# *Outlive*
# THE LABELS

## *Volume II*
## *From Trauma to Triumph*

## *VISIONARY*
### *#1 INTERNATIONAL BEST-SELLING AUTHOR*
# *MARY KAYE HOLMES*
#### *+17 Thought Leaders and Overcomers*

Outlive the Labels Volume II
From Trauma to Triumph
ISBN 978-1-5136-8374-4

Joan Tomlinson Publishing
Printed in the United States of America

# Table of Contents

# KEEP MOVING FORWARD
## FROM TRAUMA TO LIVING MY TRUTH
### MARY KAYE HOLMES

*"There is no greater agony than bearing
an untold story inside of you."*
- Maya Angelou

*E*very one of us has a story. Some of us have been through some unimaginable, unbearable trauma in our lives and I know what that feels like. I know what it's like to hit rock bottom and to feel as if the weight of the world is too much for you to get up and start over. At times the easiest thing to do is to give up and throw in the towel. Have you ever felt like giving up? I certainly felt like giving up many times throughout my life and my journey has not been easy. But, I'm so grateful that no matter the trauma, the setbacks, the disappointments, and the heartbreak — I kept going.

It all started when I was four years old and experienced the trauma of sexual molestation by an older male relative.

Sadly, the molestation continued throughout my early childhood years, but I was afraid to tell anyone, especially my mom, because I thought I would get into trouble. Like most children, I had no clue what was happening to me, but it embedded in me the beginnings of anxiety and I felt closed off from everyone else. I felt like an outsider and as if I never fit in anywhere and I especially felt like a misfit within my own family.

I didn't fit in at school either. I recall in my elementary school years I struggled to fit in with the "cool kids." My mom couldn't afford to buy me the latest sneakers and clothes, so I was often made fun of for the way I dressed. I had a thick, southern accent and was constantly teased for the way I spoke. The bullying, the fights with both girls and boys, the name calling, and the teasing from my own siblings crushed what little self-esteem I had. The shame, humiliation, and embarrassment caused me to go from being a talkative, bubbly, energetic young eight, nine, and ten-year-old girl to becoming a soft spoken, fearful, introvert.

Imagine breaking free from the childhood sexual abuse and boldly expressing all that you are only to have it beaten back inside of you. Imagine constantly being told to shut up and experiencing the sting of rejection so young. Now, imagine how relieved I was when young boys started noticing me and instead of rejecting me they *wanted* me. The compliments and the attention from the boys in my fifth and sixth grade class made me feel desirable, but there was still something missing. Several of my female classmates were already having sex and it felt almost impossible to compete with the more experienced girls. Their bodies were more developed, they dressed in see-through blouses, cropped tops, and biker shorts, and they knew how to flirt with boys in a way that my shyness would not allow. Yet, in spite of my underdeveloped figure and my quirky ways, the boys still chased after me. I was too young to know what they really wanted, but by the time I figured it out I had lost my virginity at 12 and by the time I reached 14 years old I was pregnant.

It was during that time that I became infatuated with a 16-year-old boy in my high school. We dated for a few months and eventually started having sex. It felt exciting, liberating, and a welcomed distraction from the chaos going on at home. At the time, my mom and her husband had separated after he became an alcoholic and heavily addicted to crack. The issues they experienced in the marriage caused my mom to live life in a fog of long work days, church services, and hours on the phone trying to sort out her personal life. It didn't help that I was the youngest in my family, so by the time I was in high school my mom often allowed me to freely come and go. It was as if she had grown tired of trying to keep me under control. Back then, 14 felt like adulthood in between the partying, weed smoking, and sex. I was a rebellious teen looking to outrun a quickly approaching wave of depression.

Meanwhile, my boyfriend and I thought we would be together forever. After getting pregnant we made plans to raise our child and finish high school together. We were confident that we could eventually balance college life and parenthood. We sat around for hours after school planning our future and thinking of names for our unborn baby. Sadly, when we broke the news to our parents my mother forced me get an abortion. I was devastated! What little excitement I had about life became suffocated with sadness and shortly after the abortion I attempted suicide for the first time. I locked myself in a bathroom and swallowed a bottle full of pills in an effort to escape my shattered life. Not long afterwards, my relationship with my boyfriend fizzled out and I watched helplessly as other girls captured his attention. I felt defeated.

There I was, an emotional wreck, sitting on the sidelines while the more mentally stable and more confident girls drew him further and further away from me. At the time, I didn't know how to work through the emotional pain of a surgical abortion. To have my hopes and dreams ripped and scraped out of me like trash to be discarded made me feel helpless, useless, and lonely — especially when the relationship disintegrated shortly after losing our baby. I went from watching my belly slowly swell with a life that I created with my first love to seeing it sink back down to a flattened nothing. One can imagine that at the tender age of 14 I didn't know how to unpack my emotional baggage. Instead, I just sat under the weight of it all.

I was vulnerable, impressionable, and ripe for the taking. The following year, at the age of 15, I met a 36-year-old man who took advantage of my brokenness and slowly groomed me into human trafficking. He would come to my job and flirt with me and pull out stacks of folded cash and slowly peel off a $20 bill to pay for his $2.50 smoothie. He was flashy and definitely had the gift of gab. One day, in between the flirting and the fast talking, he said something to me that would change my world forever. "How would you like to make more money in one day than you can make in an entire week working on this job?" he said. I took the bait and the rest was history. For seven long years I was trapped, brain washed, and abused by this man. It became even harder to escape once he isolated me from my family and turned me against almost everyone that I loved.

I'm grateful that I eventually escaped after seven years, but the human trafficking and the domestic abuse took a major toll on me. My self-esteem was destroyed, anxiety took over my emotions, and I constantly felt like a failure. When I looked back over my life I realized that my childhood had been stolen from me. My early 20s blew past me in a blur and I witnessed old high school friends graduate from college, get married, and move forward with their lives. Yet, there I was, stuck in my past with tons of potential but nothing to show for it. I was always the smart girl and people had high expectations for me, but I slowly shrank back until I was nearly invisible.

One day, I decided to step out of the shadows of trauma and live in my truth. My life suddenly shifted from the girl with potential to the potent powerhouse I am today when I became unapologetic about my past and asked God to deliver me from trauma. The same person who constantly procrastinated and hesitated as a result of years of intimidation by her abuser, dramatically changed course all because of a decision. I decided to put my shoulders back, stand up, and show up. I decided to dust myself off, start over, and move forward. I decided that education was going to be my key to transformation, so I reenrolled in college and got my Associates Degree. I decided to keep going and I earned my Bachelor's in Psychology. I still wasn't satisfied so I applied to law school, earned my Juris Doctorate, and passed the bar on my first attempt.

I now serve as In-House Counsel for an insurance and investments firm in New York City. When I was offered this prestigious position, I was told that it's almost unheard of for first year lawyers to land a job like mine. However, it was because of my faith, my determination, my persistence, and my ability to see myself beyond my current condition that allowed me to be where I am today. Where I was didn't determine who I was. At times I felt myself sinking back into depression, but I reminded myself to keep moving forward because there was someone coming behind me that needed to see me cross the finish line. Even if I had to desperately crawl and claw my way over, I needed to finish. This has always been bigger than me!

This is why I share my story. This is why I am bold and transparent about my truth. Maya Angelou once said, "there is no greater agony than bearing an untold story inside of you." Don't die with your story buried on the inside! Someone's life is depending on you opening up, speaking up, standing up, and showing up for them. They need to witness your strength and tenacity because it will give them the power to own their voice, and not just own it, but use it as well. Who loses out when you shrink back? Who misses out when you refuse to share your message? Break out, break free, and take back your truth — it's your story!

# BREAK FREE FROM FEAR

Are you holding your untold story hostage because of the fear of criticism, backlash, or failure? Maybe you're afraid that people won't believe you or won't accept you as a result of sharing your pain. Or maybe you have a fear that when you finally speak up no one will be there to listen. However, you have to kill this fear because it is only holding you back from breaking free. There is an invisible wall in front of you called fear and it is the only barrier between you and your next level. I'm going to share with you three strategies that I've learned over the years that helped me overcome the apprehension and the intimidation I felt when I first became transparent about my truth.

1. **Know your "why."** When you understand why you want to share your story it can be fuel to that flickering fire inside of you. Instead of that fire dying out, it rapidly spreads and becomes hard to extinguish because you become motivated by a mission.

   Do you want to share your story to touch lives and ultimately change them? Do you want to change laws? Do you want to empower women? Do you want to move people to a specific action? Do you want to motivate audiences to overcome their own fears and step out on faith?

   Maybe you're like me and you want to increase

awareness surrounding a specific cause like human trafficking or domestic violence. Ask yourself why you want to share your story and boldly stand behind it.

2. **See it before it happens.** I often use the power of my subconscious mind to overcome fear and doubt. Whenever I have a major goal ahead of me that I want to accomplish, I imagine myself already having done the very thing that I desire. Before I ever spoke on a stage or ever held a microphone and told my story, I saw myself on major platforms. I saw myself speaking to an audience of thousands. I saw myself being interviewed on television and publishing multiple books. I not only saw it, but I started speaking what I saw.

   Use the power of your subconscious mind to overcome your fear of speaking up and owning your truth. Start telling yourself that you are free from fear and that you are open and bold about sharing your story. Picture yourself holding a microphone, speaking on a stage, and confidently conveying your message. Now do it.

   Walk around your living room speaking as if you have a full audience. Speak to yourself in the mirror. Record yourself speaking. Do whatever you can to get the words out of your head and out in the open. When you're ready, record a video for social media or go live. Tell your testimony at your church or share your story in a small group setting. Whatever it takes, just start speaking. It's your voice, so use it!

3.  **Sharing your story is a part of the healing process.** When you speak up, you not only heal yourself, but you help others heal as well. You overcome by the words of your testimony, your story. The beauty in the overcoming is that you are no longer stuck within the confines of your past and you become bigger than what happened to you.

    Yes, you may have experienced some setbacks in life and made some horrendous mistakes. Yes, some of the trauma was self-inflicted. Yes, everyone may have witnessed you falling flat on your face, but there is still a fight left in you. The fact that you picked up this book and decided to read it proves that there is still a fight left in you. The very fact that you are still breathing proves that there is still a fight left in you. And because you still have a fight there is still time to finish, and the journey has only begun. Welcome to your first day of freedom. I can't wait to hear your story.

Dr. Mary Kaye Holmes is a #1 International Best-Selling Author and has authored eight books. She is a Certified Life Coach, International Speaker, Pastor, Podcaster, and Editor-in-Chief of *Style & Grace Magazine.* Her podcast

*Outlive the Labels* is featured in over twelve countries and available on Spotify, Apple Podcasts, Google Podcasts, iHeart Radio, Pandora and many other platforms.

Mary Kaye has dedicated her life to helping others by launching "Outlive the Labels" — a global movement with a mission to spread awareness of human trafficking, support survivors of trauma, and amplify the voices of those unknown, unseen, and unheard. Through collaborative book projects, she empowers survivors to share, write, and publish their stories and many of them become authors for the first time. She serves as a mentor for at-risk teen girls alongside the Chef Jeff Project and through her private mentorship programs as well.

To support and stay updated on new projects you can follow Mary Kaye on all social media platforms @hearmaryspeak and visit marykayeholmes.com where you will find her first memoir *Stripped: A Journey from Rejection to Redemption* and latest book *Trapped in Plain Sight: The Unfamiliar Face of Human Trafficking*.

Dr. Mary Kaye is a graduate of New York Law School and currently serves as In-House Counsel for a NYC insurance and investments firm. She resides in New York with her supportive husband.

Want to co-author the next volume of "Outlive the Labels"? Email info@marykayeholmes.com to get started today!

# LIVING ON THE BACKSIDE OF BETTER
## KENYA FRAZIER

*Philippians 4:12-13, "I know how to be abased and I know how to abound."*

It is with somber reflection that I think back to that day in September 2012. I was 5' 7" and 283 pounds. There I lay, sobbing on the bathroom floor, head hung low, both hands covering my face. I was in despair as my 3-year-old daughter and 13-year-old son, stood aghast. My children had just witnessed the tail-end of a fight between me and my husband. He stood 6' 3" tall and approximately 240 pounds. As we tussled back and forth, I almost lost my footing and fell backwards in the tub. It was by God's grace that I didn't fall or wasn't physically injured that day. The wounds on the inside increased with every exchange of blows. Our contempt for each other intensified.

There in that bathroom, as I lay on the floor the bombardment of derogatory epithets further confirmed that I was in a toxic relationship. The words echoed loudly in my ear: "You dumb b****!" "Shut up you fat b****!" My children were paralyzed with fear. Their silence was so loud. I was too embarrassed to look them in the eye envisioning the impact of trauma they experienced by witnessing domestic violence. My son, 13 years old at the time, had a range of emotions. I could feel his sadness and anger. The look in his eyes showed me that he wanted take matters into his own hands however intimidation prevailed. He put one hand on my shoulder gently. Too embarrassed to face him, I fixated my gaze to the ground. His voice cracked as he asked, "Are you okay mom?" I responded, "Yes, Chris. Mommy is okay." My 3-year-old daughter looked at me with concern. She had one hand holding her favorite sippy cup and with the other, she grabbed my hand and said, "Come on Mommy! I'll help you up."

That was one of the lowest moments I had ever experienced. The culmination of disrespect, degradation, humiliation, and violence had taken its toll. I felt reduced to nothing in front of my children. I said to myself, "Kenya, you are unloved, disliked and lonely as a wife and failing as a mother." I wanted so badly to get up off that bathroom floor and re-assure my children that home would be a better, safer place, but I couldn't. I describe my situation as living on the backside of better. Mine was a life of discordance and incongruencies. Living on the backside of better I experienced prosperity coupled with calamity. Having children, an education, and a great career all while living in a beautiful community in the robust city of Charlotte, North Carolina was exhilarating. But there were many moments of displeasure as life seemed out of my control. Love was also elusive.

Feeling powerless, I was unable to create a happy home. My spouse had angry outbursts, fluctuating mood swings, and heightened anxiety. He wasn't happy and there was nothing I could do to create harmony. We engaged in a toxic exchange of yelling, cursing, and accusations. I was melancholy and regretful of the choices I made for me and my children. Anger conflated with acrimony. There were many days I was overwhelmed and had outbursts too. I was no angel. I turned into a woman I despised. I would say things to emasculate my husband. Praying often to no avail, my petition for reconciliation wasn't granted. I felt abandoned in a godforsaken place.

Back then, I dwelled on the backside of better. Every decision I made in life was to avoid being a statistic and outlive the labels. Although I avoided some labels, I encountered others. I became an angry black woman and battled imposter syndrome. I felt inadequate as a psychotherapist and subsequently closed my private practice. Being an "imposter" was too burdensome. I was empty inside, a mere shell, who became unrecognizable at 283 pounds. After years of my emotional decline, I decided to pray a different prayer. I asked God to deliver me and my children safely from this situation. God heard my prayer and He answered. God gave me a plan of escape. In 2014, I secured a contract position working as counselor on a military base in Texas. Me and my two children lived in a hotel room for three months. I wasn't allowed to take my children with me on this work assignment, but I snuck them into the hotel hoping my job wouldn't find out. I was tired, at my lowest, and on the edge. But when I told God "yes" to His plan my faith increased, and the Lord took care of the rest! My employer paid for my hotel room and flight to and from Texas. I was provided a car and a stipend for gas and meals. I made close to $2000 per week that I pocketed because my employer paid my living expenses. That was the most money I ever accumulated while working!

My life nearly came to a halt when a colleague knocked on my door and could hear my children laughing and playing. When she found out that I had them with me, she reported me to the Army Sergeant. I was devastated and prepared for the worst. Days later I was called into the office. The Sergeant called me in to notify me that my colleague was fired for displaying bizarre behavior. She also told me this colleague reported me for having my children with me. She praised my work ethic and said they wanted me there permanently, WITH MY CHILDREN! When my contract with the military ended, I moved back home to Charlotte, hired a divorce attorney, separated in 2015 and was divorced by 2016! I never looked back! The path to healing was a process. I started with focusing on my self-care. I joined a gym. I connected with loved ones. I participated in activities I loved such as shopping, pedicures, watching movies, and outings with friends. I renewed my relationship with Christ. I fasted and prayed. I wrote in my journal and engaged in counseling. My self-esteem increased by meditating on God's Word and extending gratitude. Every morning, I recited positive affirmations over my life. I re-evaluated the people in my life. I distanced myself from unsupportive "friends" and spent more time with people who genuinely loved me.

My life transformed when I found positive ways to restore my brokenness. I even became a better mother. With humility, I asked my children to forgive me for exposing them to trauma. We communicated and processed our feelings, which strengthened our bond. After becoming whole, I was further rejuvenated caring for others, specifically children in foster care. All the above actions contributed to my healing. Today, I'm thankful that God helped me overcome and triumph over this situation. Having a relationship with Christ transformed me. My quality of life has improved. My joy is restored. I own a beautiful home and live with my two children, who are my joy. I'm also a proud mom to a son in his final year of college. God has been faithful to me!

# Goals for Self-Care

*Life has its share of obstacles and adversity. Therefore, it is important to be kind to ourselves during times of challenges. Healing must be intentional. Happiness is a choice. How we present ourselves in this world and in the face of adversity has much to do with how we feel about ourselves. Make an internal commitment to show up for yourself. You cannot expect anyone to care for you more than you care for yourself. You model to others how you want to be treated by how you treat yourself. Give yourself permission to handle yourself with care. Self-care is imperative for growing and healing. For many of us self-care does not come easy, especially for those of us who feel a sense of guilt when placing attention on our own needs and desires. I have included some strategies that you can implement daily, weekly, or monthly. I wish you all the best on your journey to wellness.*

**Nourishing the Mind:**
- *Read a book*
- *Meditate*
- *Deep breathing exercise*
- *Recite positive affirmations*
- *Turn your phone off*
- *Keep a compliment notebook*
- *Don't be hard on yourself/Forgive yourself*

*Nourishing the Body:*

- *Eat a healthy meal*
- *Workout*
- *Get a massage (get hair/nails done)*
- *Drink water*
- *10-minute stretch*
- *Take a hot bath*
- *Go to bed early*

*Nourishing the Soul:*

- *Go outside, get in sunlight*
- *Volunteer/help someone in need*
- *Connect with people you love*
- *Pray, read scriptures or inspirational literature*
- *Create a vision board*
- *Tap into your creative side (poetry, singing, baking)*
- *Keep a gratitude journal*

Kenya Frazier is a Licensed Clinical Social Worker currently licensed in North Carolina and South Carolina. Ms. Frazier has over 20 years of experience in the field of social work and has had clinical licensure for over 10 years. She started her career working as a psychotherapist at a psychiatric hospital providing individual and group therapy to patients on the adult inpatient acute unit. Ms. Frazier also has experience as a Military Family and Life Counselor, providing support to active-duty military personnel and their families. She currently holds a corporate position as a LCSW and is also an independent contractor with a private practice where she offers individual therapy along with clinical supervision to provisionally licensed clinical social workers. Ms. Frazier is a divorced, mother of two and a Believer. She is a therapeutic foster mother and mentor to adolescent girls in foster care. Ms. Frazier is an advocate for women's empowerment, helping women to gain the skills needed to achieve healing from trauma, increase resilience, and overcome adversity. Aside from her professional career, Ms. Frazier loves fashion. She more recently added freelance modeling to her repertoire of talents as she models for local brands in the Charlotte area.

Website: www.kenyafrazierlcsw.com
IG: @kenya.frazier_lcsw
Email: kenyaf.lcsw@gmail.com

# SONGBIRD SOUNDS OFF
## CYNTHIA CORDERO

"*Sound off! 1,2! Sound off! 3,4! Sound off! Now bring it on down 1,2,3,4… 1,2,3,4!!!*" That was the sound of me and my girls doing our thing with our cheers. We were loud, confident and with our moves you couldn't tell us nothing! I smile thinking about all the fun I had growing up in those Brooklyn projects in spite of the challenges I faced in other parts of my life. Early on it was revealed that I could sing, and I would be asked to do it often. I sang pretty much anywhere I was asked to. At school I was a soloist for the plays and assemblies. I even sang at my aunt's church a few times. It was a great feeling to receive attention like that, although I don't think at the time I fully understood that it was a talent, a gift. As a little girl I would have my pretend microphone and be anyone I wanted, from Diana Ross to Barbra Streisand. I fantasized about becoming a star, with records and movie deals, wearing beautiful clothes and living far away from the realities I faced. In that project apartment I would sit in the hallway when I was alone and enjoy the acoustics of that space. I would sing, and no one was there to tell me to shut up, that I was annoying, that I would never make it, or that I would be nothing. I was free to be me, even though I wasn't fully sure of who I was. I knew I could sing although a part of me began to think maybe I sounded "off" and that's why some would try to silence me. Maybe I wasn't good enough?

My friends and I loved to dance so we went to audition for a talent show. While there one of my friends suggested I sing, so I did. I won the Brooklyn round and was going to city wide but was told nobody was taking me there or getting anyone to play the piano for me, so I couldn't go. I lost out time after time because "no" was what I received from those that should have been my biggest cheerleaders. When you're met with disappointments, lack of support, loss of opportunities that you earned, it begins to break you and parts of you that made you feel special and alive simply die. It seems pointless to put yourself out there if you're not going to be able to enjoy the prize. In junior high school I joined the gospel choir, which was great, and my music teacher took special interest in me. He began to train me classically, preparing me to audition for Performing Arts H.S. It was around this time that thoughts of ending it all grew louder as I now felt like I was just going through the motions. I was notified that I was chosen for a boarding school scholarship and even that meant little to the adults in my life.

Weaved into those happy, winning moments was much darkness and the glow in my eyes was becoming faint. I was still a straight-A student and I worked hard at that. I didn't talk too much about what was going on inside of me, which felt like a slow fade. There were times I just didn't want to live anymore, and I felt like I should become someone else that others would approve. This included "the boy" I met while in junior high, who became a distraction I welcomed because it helped me forget what was really looming over me. That distraction led to detours and I began to close doors. I missed more auditions including Performing Arts H.S. since I had no support and no longer bothered to ask. I was robbed time after time.

As a teen my "boyfriend" told me there was a guy looking for a singer for a project, so I went and sang again. The idea sounded good coming from him. There was a glimpse of hope for a dream I thought was gone. I enjoyed it but unfortunately, betrayal and deceit caused me to lose again. Why did I keep trying? I felt foolish. A chance taken in trusting others with my talent and heart failed me. Singing no longer felt like a good thing, so I decided it would not be a major focus. By this time my attention was not just on school, and I looked for value where it could not be found and gave power to people who could not and should not have been responsible for what was placed in their hands. I felt lost.

Still the smart, popular girl I went on to become senior class President, Salutatorian and earned all kinds of other awards but singing was not at the top of the list. It's like I was finally on mute and although the desire remained, it was dormant. I went on and resolved myself to the life I created through some poor decisions and I settled. Muffled and silenced I would watch others do what I longed for, but as time passed fear had also settled in along with the notion that it wasn't for me and that rang loud. Losing heart and experiencing hurt, that slow fade flat-lined and I not only believed every negative word that had been said along the way, I began to say them to myself! I bought the lie that I had "stage fright" and was silenced. I was a mom, a wife, and had my career so what more did I want?

The truth was deep down inside I still wanted to sing. I pushed, and I met a vocal coach, Allyson Starr who said, "My dear, it is an insult to God when we don't use our gifts and you sweetheart have an amazing gift. Now use it!" How I wish I had the chance to tell her how she blessed me. As things in my life fell apart and unfolded I went back to church. I sat and watched the singers on that pulpit and there was that feeling again. I wanted to sing with them and God set things up as only He can. He lovingly nudged me up there and suddenly there I was. While there I met a beautiful lady, who began to call me Songbird and at first, I felt funny about the name. She said it with such love and once I came to the place of truly accepting the name she gave me it did something special for me. I started taking risks and investing in myself. Those risks led to opportunities, singing with an entertainment company and meeting R&B singer Chrisette Michele who became my vocal coach and mentor. Taking steps, fighting back and finding my voice I now see who God says I am and what He has called me to be and do. I choose to believe in me when it gets hard, lonely, or when it seems as if people don't understand. I freely embrace the name and this Songbird sounds off whenever and wherever because after all, *"It Is a Gift, My Dear."*

My Dear,

Let me start by saying that you may not sing, but this still applies to you. If it hasn't, it's time for "your thing", your gift, your talent to come forth. Just like I couldn't shake off what was actually a part of me I'm sure you can't either, so it's time to connect with that part of you and make it happen! For me, devotionals, time with God, and meditating on what He said about me was and still is such a big deal in the process — the journey. Transformation is often thought of as being cute and pretty, but it can be dirty, and you must dig deep at times so be ready for that. What unfolds can be beautiful and amazing. Be ready for that too. Let's Go. Journey with Me.

- What's Your Thing? You have one, trust me. I know it's a common suggestion but write down that dream, that plan. See it on paper and keep it before you. I carried around a little book with those notes, affirmations and scriptures that helped me. It's something I do to this day along with vision boards and boxes.

- Intentionally set aside space where you can create, pray and just be... remember to rest.

- Fear is paralyzing, and I ask that you don't let it keep you bound for years like I did. Acknowledge it, face it head on, and replace it with faith. Kick it all the way out the door because it can't stay. Know that this will be something you do consistently.

- Speak now or forever let someone or something hold your peace and your purpose. Take ownership of them. Speak those things that you are believing for yourself no matter how big they seem. Speak your peace into place because you will need it to continue the journey, especially when naysayers show up and they may be people you really love. Do not agree with the negativity and the lies. Say you can even when a thought that you can't creeps in. It's okay to talk to yourself.

- Speaking of letting someone hold your peace, forgiveness of yourself and others is crucial to the journey. I'll leave this part with the request that you consider who and what came to mind when you read this point and what you should do next.

- Find out who's got your six — who's got your back. Sometimes your circle changes and you have to be good with that. I fought this part to the point of tears and it didn't help me. Let it go! You have work to do anyway and those who want to see you win will show up. They will challenge you and love on you when necessary. I had another vocal coach who forced me to sing at a karaoke spot in front of a bunch of people I didn't know to get over that "stage fright." We are friends to this day.

- Invest in you. You're worth it. The idea of making certain investments was not a concept I embraced at first, but it is necessary. I required coaches and I had and still have to invest time and money into my journey. When you realize your purpose is important and people are attached to it, who need what you have, it becomes a priority.

- Arise! Emerge! It's your time to shine!
- Do it afraid! Sound Off! Open your mouth and find your voice. The world is waiting!

*"And when she thought her life was over she transformed and unfolded perfectly."*
- Dr. Cynthia Cordero "Dr. Cee Cee"

Cynthia Cordero, a graceful force in the Kingdom of God, is first a proud mom of two and grandmother to an adorable little girl. Cynthia is a retired NYPD Detective who was deemed a specialist in her assignment with youth and community. She is also a 9/11 WTC Responder. She now works in the SDNY Federal Courts under the USMS. Cynthia is a Chaplain and UN Peace Ambassador serving also as Deputy Director General of the Security Department for the International Consulting Cabinet of WOLMI. She is a Not on My Watch advocate against domestic violence and human trafficking and is a Director of the Brooklyn unit.

Cynthia is a speaker, vocalist, certified life transformation coach and host of EmergeNCee Break! Podcast. As a bestselling author she has made contributions to amazing projects such as *Outlive the Labels*, *Victim to Victory*, and *Oh Mari!* a children's book series. She is also the founder of the Mari Movement dedicated to combat bullying and youth suicide — a cause she took on after losing her niece to this evil.

Cynthia attends Overflow Christian Center where she serves in the Children and Teen Ministry, sings on the Praise and Worship Team and is President of the Dream Girl Women's Ministry. She owns and operates CC Conglomerate LLC and Mariposa Ministries.

www.cynthiacordero.com
Facebook – Cynthia Cordero
IG - @drcynthiacordero

# ASSET-TUDE & STRATEGIC SELFISHNESS
## MADAME PEONY

*asset-tude* is a personal construction not found in a dictionary. It means recognizing that money is not confetti. It is an important tool for education, personal growth, future security, and pleasure in life. *Strategic selfishness* is thinking about the effect of hasty generosity to your *asset-tude* goals (if you have none, make some). The following episodes from my own life illustrate how ignorance of *asset-tude* and *strategic selfishness* led me to make the same mistake that would total $1,600 over 40 years. The sum is not important, it is the hurt, helplessness, and embarrassment that never quite go away.

I went into the military as soon as I graduated high school. Four dollars an hour was the most I had ever made from part-time jobs so my monthly pay—at a little over $400 a month—seemed like a fortune. I had a lot more experience with not having money. My mother struggled to support her children, and sometimes failed to keep a roof over our heads. When money came in, it was already owed, or just enough to cover basic needs. She had also grown up poor and did not have *asset-tude* to teach me.

My home training revolved around being a nice person, being respectful to adults, and being responsible for my brother and sisters. I was taught to clean the house by nine years old and to cook before I was a teenager. Mama knew that not every friend, relative or stranger was to be trusted, but she never passed that lesson onto me.

When I was eleven, I spent the summer with family who lived out of state. My teenaged cousin took me to visit a girl she knew. I do not remember the conversation that revealed my possession of my $5 weekly allowance, but her friend asked to 'borrow' it. I did not know what to do. I had been raised to be nice and I thought I was doing the "nice" thing. My cousin's friend never paid me back. The last time I saw her, she was defiant, challenging, and said, "I just don't have it," knowing there was nothing I could do. I went home with hurt feelings, but no wiser from the experience.

In 1976, America was high on our Bicentennial year, but my boyfriend was lower than sewer sludge. He borrowed the money I was saving for my Mother's Day gift, then ducked me for the rest of the school year. Two years later, I was in the military. An Airman in my training class came to me, in tears, with a hard luck story about a family crisis. He needed to borrow $400. Shortly thereafter he was showing off the expensive camera he bought with my money. When I appealed to our commanding officer, he asked me if I had 'proof' that I 'loaned' him the money. I was a nice person. I trusted his story, but without proof he said there was nothing he could do. But even today, the hurt on my soul reminds me that he did not give a damn.

The next time, I could not blame the inexperience of youth. I was in my 40s when I loaned my "best friend" $1,200. My skeptical husband smirked as he told me, "You know, you're never getting that money back." "Oh no," I insisted. "She'll pay me back." I was sure because we were friends for over 10 years. This was the most money I had loaned anyone before and the only time I ever had that much money to loan. I have needed that money several times over the years, but the friend was going through her own difficulties and I did not have the heart to ask. I did receive one payment of $50 two years ago…that was the first and last.

Did I learn from previous experience? Well, yes *and* no. A co-worker and friend I affectionately call, "My Personal White Dude", would borrow small sums, $5, $7, $10. I never kept track. When I called in his debts, I thought the sum was more than he thought owed. I insisted, and he paid, but it was not a happy settlement. The next time he needed a loan, I printed out a contract that included a statement about him owing me his blood if he did not pay me back. He returned my money the next day, admitting that my "blood clause" made him nervous. I had finally discovered the key to repayment, but it may only work with Catholics.

I hope *asset-tude* and *strategic selfishness* will save others from making my bad judgements. I never want to read another story like the one that ran in 2011 under the New York Post headline, "Brooklyn Woman Kills Brother's Girlfriend Over $20." At 22 she was dead because of a $20 loan for a pack of diapers.

## Develop *"asset-tude"*

When people know you have money, they know where to go when they need money. Keep your assets to yourself.

- Your winning lottery ticket is nobody's business.
- Your salary or legal settlement are nobody's business.
- Your birthday money or inheritance are nobody's business.
- Your holiday bonus or tax refund are nobody's business.

However, when someone asks to borrow *your* money, they make their business your affair. Ask questions, pay attention, and make notes. Later think about their answers. Did their story sound realistic or shady? Were they consistent and clear? Did they show you any proof? Did you feel they are being honest? Were they offended or irritated by your questions—this may reveal future problems. Set clear expectations so there is no confusion.

*These are sample questions, but ask others relevant to your situation:*

- What is the loan for?
- Can I make a direct payment (for a bill or rent)? Why not?
- Will you sign a contract?
- Do you have collateral?
- How will you pay me back?

- Can you pay me back by___? (set a date within 3 months because people have short memories).

## *Strategic selfishness in decision-making:*

Listen, but do not commit. "I'm not ready to make a decision," is a good response.

- Do not be manipulated by guilt or pressure.
- Do not loan to liars, irresponsible, or difficult people.
- Do not loan your savings, rent, or other expenses.
- Do not loan to people who owe you money.
- Never make a loan with an open-ended date: set a firm date, period.
- Do not loan more than you can lose—you may never be repaid.
- Do not make a loan without a contract.
- Do not make a loan dependent on a settlement or tax return—that money may be spent before you know they had it.

If you do not want to loan this person money, say, "This is a bad time." You owe no one an explanation. And in the future, you may be able to do them a different favor. There are people who deserve help, but not everyone deserves equally.

But if you want to help someone and avoid a headache: give anonymously. Your relationship might be better that way.

# CONTRACT

I _____ (name of borrower)

agree to pay _____ (name of lender)

$_____ (amount of the loan) for _____ (reason for loan)

by _____ (date to be repaid). I understand that by signing this

document, I am signing a legally binding contract.


_____     _____

Name of borrower    Date    Name of lender    Date

...........

If the loan is being paid in installments add:

I agree to pay in_____(number of installments) on
_____(dates of repayment)

...........

If the loan is secured with collateral add:

I understand if I do not repay this load as agreed in this contract
the _____ (describe the collateral) will become
the property of _____name of lender.


(Both parties sign 2 original copies. Each person receives a
copy. If the agreement changes, a new contract with the
changes must be made and signed. Must be 18 years or older
to enter a contract without a parent or guardian.)

Madame Peony, a native of Greenville, SC was raised in
Brooklyn, NY. She did stage work in her teens in the youth

theatres, "Of, By & For" and StageWorks, associated with Long Island University. In the 1990s she founded Black Community Arts Books (BCA) which had locations in New Brunswick, NJ and Philadelphia, PA. As a textile artist she exhibited at Weeksville, NY, Princeton, NJ and Plainsboro, NJ. As "Mo Fleming" she has been published in Crab Orchard Review, written for QBR: The Black Book Review, Mosaic Magazine, Lilith: The Independent Magazine for Jewish Women, and Jareeda: The International Magazine for Middle Eastern Dance. As "Kush Miri", she is the author of a memoir, "Seasons in Sheol: My Nightmare Journey Through Synagogue Culture." She is developing a Blog to help youths navigate life, anticipated to start fall of 2022. Madame Peony lives with her family in Bear, DE.

# LIFE AFTER DEATH
## KIM DAWSON

"*H*e's not getting better, Hon." Those were the words-my sister in law, Beverly, spoke to me over the phone. In my mind I told myself, "*Oh he's just going to be in a coma a little while longer*" but my heart told me the truth... that he was gone!

Ten days prior, I had just turned thirty, now I was a widow - a word that was foreign to me, a disgusting ugly word. A LABEL that I didn't want to accept. It was as if I was Hester Prynne from *The Scarlet Letter*, only I was condemned to wear a Giant W on my chest for the rest of my life. All the widows that I had known were women older in age or women I had read about in the Bible. I certainly didn't know any thirty-year-old, childless widows. At the age of thirty, I had not suffered any major losses in my family. I still had my parents and all my siblings. Up until this point my greatest fear had been losing my mother who had been terminally ill with kidney disease. But my mother hadn't died, it was my newly wedded husband, my friend and my lover of only two years and nine months.

At that moment I was thrust into a grief that was so consuming that I thought that at any moment I would perish myself. It wasn't just my heart that was broken but it was my entire being. It was like I felt a searing, burning pain throughout my body. I physically felt that the two who had once become one flesh were now being separated. Now imagine going into surgery with no anesthesia to have a limb removed. Imagine the searing or the tearing of flesh and how that might feel. Not pleasant!

The homegoing was beautiful from what I can remember. However, what I distinctively recall is, my two best friends carrying me to the car after the repass. They opened the back door and I collapsed, sobbing in the back seat. It was done!! I had carried out one of the most sacred and important tasks in my life, I had buried my husband and it was done! I'm not sure at what moment it happened, but it happened. I stopped living and that was the biggest mistake that I made during my grief process. My grief became depression. I stopped going to work, I left my home, put it up for sale and moved back in my childhood bedroom.

Sleep escaped me, and food just didn't taste good any more. I was now doing more damage to my mind and body than the grief. I now know, that sleep deprivation brings on delirium. The less sleep we have, the less we're able to function. I was also starving my brain and body of necessary nutrients that help to build up necessary hormones like serotonin and other brain chemicals. I was in the deep throngs of depression; I was a train wreck waiting to happen. I couldn't pray a substantial prayer because my brain wasn't functioning properly BUT as the song goes, somebody prayed for me! I thank God for the prayers of the righteous! I had the best support team that anyone could ask for. Not just my family, but my church family, my lifelong friends and even collogues at work. I'm not sure if she knows it or not but my boss saved my life. After stalling and not returning to work for about 30 days, (yes, I know crazy right) I received a phone call from my supervisor, Kathy. She didn't threaten to take my job, nor did she ask when, she just said, "Kim you have to come back to work." It was as if I was a little child waiting for someone to tell me what to do. She beckoned, and I agreed. That was the beginning of healing.

That Monday morning, I shed tears the whole time that I was getting dressed, I didn't want to face the world because of the label that I carried, WIDOW. I prayed with every step that I took and made it through the day, then I made it through another day and then another. However, I was still not myself. I was in such depression and despair, BUT the difference now was, I wanted out of the black hole. I didn't know how to get out. Then I made a decision and did something that is taboo in both the black church and community. I decided that I would go to therapy. Ironically, my therapist was an educated man of his craft, Pastor and man of God. It was no mistake at all and it ended up being one of the best decisions I ever made.

Slowly, day by day, I began to come out of my black hole. I began exercising and eating right under the guidance of my best friend and personal trainer, Vania. Prayer and meditation become part of my daily schedule again. Then I made the PERSONAL choice to take medication. Yes! I took medication under the supervision of my therapist and family doctor. I realize that this is another stigma and not a decision that everyone will feel is right for them, but it was right for me. My doctor explained that after being depressed for so long your brain is depleted of important hormones, the happy hormones, and it sometimes need a kick start. Can I tell you what a difference it made for me! I remember the first day I began taking it. My colleagues and I had a training in Wethersfield, CT for work and decided to carpool. I specifically choose the back seat all to myself. Can I tell you I got in the back seat and sleep all the way there and back! That's how exhausted my body was, and I didn't even realize it. My co-worker later told me "I knew you were tired and needed rest, so I just let you sleep" and not only did she let me sleep but she also prayed for me.

Therapy, prayer, exercise, rest and medication all contributed to my healing and brought me back to life. I remember a month after beginning my regimen, I was leaving my appointment and the sun was shining so bright and I could see it and it was beautiful! I could feel the warmth as it beamed down on me and the gentle spring breeze as it blew, and it felt good. I could feel again, I was alive, happy to be alive and enjoying being alive.

Grief is a part of life and its okay to grieve but how we grieve is important. I'm reminded of a line from a poem of an Unknown Author: *"So grieve a while for me, if grieve you must. Then let your grief be comforted by trust."* Fast forward to now… I can't tell you that I lived happily ever after, but I can tell you I outlived the label. I had some more great losses, I shed a lot more tears, but I learned how to grieve and heal appropriately. My grief became comforted by trust in GOD. Most importantly, I decided to live and not die!

# Activity for the Reader

| | |
|---|---|
| **G** | Give<br><br>Give your grief to God. Realize that throughout your grief God is always there with you. He understands what you are going through and cares for you. |
| **R** | Rest<br><br>Make sure you get the proper rest. Rest is not only good for your physical being but your mental being as well; it gives you clarity of thought. |
| **I** | Integrate<br><br>Integrate; don't isolate from family and friends who love you. Get out as much as you can and keep up your routines as much as possible. |
| **E** | Exercise<br><br>Take care of your physical being as well as your spiritual and mental being. Exercise releases those important chemicals that our brain needs to stay healthy. Not only will you feel better mentally but you may lose a few pounds and begin to feel better about your self-image, boosting your self-esteem and mood. |
| **V** | Validate<br><br>Validate your feelings and recognize that it's okay. Grief is a process, a process that does not necessarily go in organized steps. That's why it's important to validate what you are feeling. Realize it's okay to feel what you're feeling and keep it moving. |
| **E** | Evolve<br><br>Evolve into the new you! Whether you lost a husband or a parent, that loss caused you to become a new person so establish new routines and roles. If you were a wife, you are now a single widow. If you lost a parent, you now have to navigate life without a parent and assume the role of matriarch or patriarch. Whatever the life change is, embrace it and evolve into your new normal. |

Kim Dawson a native of Bridgeport, CT is a divorced, once widowed single mother of three boys. She is a Co-Author, Educator, Licensed Foster mother and former Program Director of ReFocus Outreach Ministries.

Through these various roles she has been the vehicle that God has used to educate countless children, usher hundreds of women out of homelessness and drug addiction, and a mother to the motherless. It is her desire to be the catalyst that God uses to propel the hopeless to hope.

Kim can be reached at kimdgibbs@gmail.com,
Facebook: Kim Dawson or Instagram: Cocoakimm.

# I CAN'T? I WILL!
## ANTOINETTE STEPHENS

*I*t was my junior year in high school. The only thing that came across my mind was, *"Where do I go from here? I only have one more year left, and I feel like a complete failure."*

After hearing it in so many words throughout the years by my teachers, how could I not think of myself any differently. By the way, my name is Antoinette Stephens and the only thing I ever wanted to do since childhood was become a lawyer or a researcher in Criminal Justice. However, I knew that with my grades I would never have the chance to accomplish my childhood dreams and the negative comments from my teachers only reaffirmed this belief.

One day I had a meeting with a teacher and she wanted to talk to me about the horrible grades I was getting and all the trouble that I brought to myself. Ms. K asked me one question, "Antoinette, what do you see in your future?" I responded, "Ms. K, I've always been interested in criminal justice research or criminal law." I had never really discussed what I wanted out of life with anyone because I was afraid of criticism. I just knew that my dreams and desires were going to be laughed at and to no surprise, Ms. K did exactly what I knew she would do — she chuckled. "What's so funny?" I asked.

"Antoinette, with your grades and all the trouble you've been getting yourself into, the closest you'll ever get to the criminal justice system is getting arrested," she said. "Hopefully that does not happen. You may need to take up a trade because no university or law school is ever going to accept you." I was hurt by her words, but I was not shocked at all. No one could understand me. I wanted to accomplish my dreams in life, but at that time, my focus seemed to not be on school. I knew teachers probably thought that I didn't have a clue on how to do anything, but that definitely wasn't the case at all. All I knew was I wanted to get somewhere in life but didn't know how to get there.

It was spring 2001, and I was attending Norwalk Community College for Criminal Justice. I didn't feel too excited, I should've been more enthusiastic, but something felt strange. I looked around the halls and stood there zoned out for about fifteen minutes wondering, *"Why am I here?"* All I could think about was all the times that I had been told that I was wasting my time and that I would not be able to do it. I was driving myself crazy, letting all these scenarios take over my mind. I finally was able to move and head to my first class. I walked in and saw so many happy faces, they were so excited to start this new journey in their lives. Not me! I sat at the desk in the corner, isolating myself from the rest of the class.

"Hello class, my name is Professor Smith, and I want to welcome everyone to Intro to Criminal Justice." Still, no excitement from me. Professor Smith seemed like an alright person; you can tell she was really into what she did. She was not going to let us leave her class without knowing what we needed to know about the criminal justice system. Professor Smith passed out a getting to know you form. One of the questions on the form stated: "What part of the field of Criminal Justice interests you?" I didn't quite know how to answer that question any longer. Every time someone asked me the question of what I wanted out of life, what I wanted to do with my life, or anything that had to do with my life, it was always laughed at or discouraged, so I never answered those types of questions anymore. I left that question blank, but I answered the rest, which was the basics that she probably knew already. I knew for a fact that this semester was not going to go well, or any semester after that. Needless to say, I was absolutely correct. After my first two semesters at Norwalk Community College, I failed out horribly. I let myself down; I just never could shake off how much of a failure I was. Well at least that's what I had been told by others. Well, I proved them right once again!

By the summer of 2012, all those years had passed me by and I hadn't accomplished anything I wanted to do in my life. I let everyone's negativity get the best of me. But, I wasn't raised that way! I was always told I can do whatever I want, as long as I remained focused. But instead I listened to people that I hardly knew. So, I enrolled back into Norwalk Community College for the second time. I was still doubting myself, but it was something about those eleven years that passed that made me feel different than I did in 2001.

I met with my advisor Mrs. Clayborn and she was a breath of fresh air. We went over my grades from 2001 and she informed me that this time around would be my time to shine I've never heard any of my teachers say anything like that to me before. It was just something about her, that made me believe that I would go further. From that day of meeting Mrs. Clayborn, she was always on me. Anytime I had issues she was there and whenever I needed tutoring she showed me how to get it. She was like my educational fairy godmother!

Well guess what? I received my Associates in Criminal justice! I was super excited! Not only did I make myself happy, I made my family happy. Mrs. Clayborn was so proud of me as well, she even helped me apply to the University of Bridgeport to further my education. Fall of 2014, the banner read welcome to the University of Bridgeport. I was so exhilarated! I was on my way! I received my Bachelor's in Criminal Justice in 2017 and my Master's in Criminal Justice in 2019. I'm two semesters away from receiving my Master of Business Administration. Mrs. Clayborn played a major part in what I have accomplished thus far, and she is still in my life after so many years.

Never let anyone dictate your future! Finding that one person like I have found that encouraged me and pushed me because she knew I had it in me, was all I needed. The girl that always felt she couldn't do it, is now doing it! What's next? Doctorate or Juris Doctorate. Thanks for believing in me, Professor Clayborn!

Hailing from Stamford, Connecticut, Antoinette Stephens is a dedicated student of her studies and has many career plans for her future. She has been on the education journey for many years and still is not done yet. With so many ups and downs, and not many people believing in her, Antoinette is on a mission to conquer everything that she was told she couldn't have. Antoinette has received her BA and MA in Criminal Justice and Human Security and is now months away from receiving her MBA, with a concentration in management. She will be furthering her education journey towards law school, in pursuit of becoming an entertainment lawyer.

# I'M TELLING MY STORY!

## JESSICA MOJICA

"Tu no sirbe para na!" "Tu eres estupida!" "Nunca ascendera a nada!" Translated in English: "You are worth nothing!" "You are stupid!" "You will never amount to anything!" There were many other words spoken, but they would take up a whole book to write.

I became a product of what I experienced and what I saw growing up. The negative words that were spoken over my life became word curses. My whole life was nothing but a catastrophe. Everything I experienced and went through led me to become a rebellious child at an early age. I had parents who had a hard time expressing love; therefore, I never received love from them or felt loved by them, and I never heard the words "I love you." I can't really blame them because they experienced a lack of love from their own parents. This became a generational curse and a cycle that passed on. My neighborhood in Brooklyn, NY is where it all started for me.

Rejection, fighting, anger, and emotional and physical abuse were at the center of my upbringing. Rejection came from parents, teachers, friends, and classmates. It also came from being bullied, molested, and raped. My identity suffered a crisis, and I developed a mindset of feeling shameful, insecure, and embarrassed. It caused me to hide, and not just physically, as I preferred not to be seen or to engage with others emotionally, but I also hid my pain from all the traumatic experiences. This caused me to rebel and go on a mission to further hurt myself by using drugs, drinking, and smoking weed. I neglected and abused my body by having sex with boys because I wanted to feel accepted. I also engaged in everything from cutting and slicing my arms, to dabbling in witchcraft, to having physical fights, to hurting people and family, to robbing, to feeling worthless and helpless and not loving myself, to putting myself into life-threatening situations. A root of bitterness, anger, and unforgiveness took a deep seat at the core of my heart. I developed a defense mechanism where I brought up walls for protection by not allowing anyone into my world.

Too much negativity clouded my mind, so my mind developed a negative belief system of lies from the enemy. I had adopted the belief that I was a nobody. I was very shy; I did not talk or smile. Everybody around me, including my family and friends, used to tease me and make fun of me. I frequently heard them say, "Why are you so serious?" I hated those words! As if I didn't know that I wasn't a happy camper like they were! They just had to push me further into my misery by asking me that. It caused me to pull away, shut down, and feel shameful. Even now, in my adult years, I still hear those words, but now I've learned not to pay them any mind or to allow them to have an effect on me. I just brush them away. The enemy always uses people to try to make me stumble.

I even experienced great rejection from my parents. I was 15 years old when I became pregnant and miscarried my baby. After rushing to the hospital with my mom in so much pain and agony, I was left in the hospital all alone miscarrying my baby because my mom left me to go visit her boyfriend who was in jail. I thank God He sent an angel nurse to hold my hand and to cry with me. To make matters worse, my father molested me at a very early age, which lasted for a few years. Not knowing who it was creeping in the middle of the night violating my innocence, I became so fearful when it happened. I hid my face under the covers, so I wouldn't see the boogie man's face.

It wasn't until later, in my mid 30s, that God revealed to me in an open vision who the boogie man was that had crept into my room. No wonder our relationship was stale and distant. The molestation affected me later on in life with men in general because I had issues trusting men. I even considered God to be untrustworthy, but I didn't realize this until God shed light on my thinking. Not only was I molested by my father, but a major drug dealer who claimed to be my friend raped me in the back of a cab; he paid the cab driver to leave the cab as he held me captive in the back seat and raped me.

In 1998, I gave my life to the Lord and it was a wonderful experience. I felt free and alive! I grew and matured with the Lord. As years went by, the Lord told me, "Jessica, there are things we're going to have to deal with — things from your past that are rooted deep within, and you don't even know they are there." He told me, "Because you've been hurt so much and have multiple wounds and trauma to your soul, my healing and deliverance process will be slow because I am very sensitive."

During the process of my healing, there were many prophetic words spoken over me concerning my calling. It was not until I came into agreement with the prophetic words and gave God a "yes" that my whole world turned upside down! God began to bring things up from the depth of my heart to deal with the issues I carried inside. He did it by using imperfect people and circumstances. It's funny how God used the very thing from my past to cause me to walk into my purpose. God had it all planned out! He deliberately brought people into my life with dysfunctional behavior to catapult me to the very thing I did not receive when I was young —love. God was looking for me to humble myself to allow the change to happen in me first. I've learned in my journey that the pain, the frustration, the discomfort, and the anger were things God was using to perfect His love in me for others. He was teaching me how to love even the most difficult of people.

When I gave God a yes, He took me through a pruning purification process before He allowed me to walk in my calling. It took me years to come out of my wilderness of negativity about myself because I was so full of shame, insecurity, bitterness, and unforgiveness. I did not love myself or others, and I was angry all the time. Too much negativity was deposited in me which clouded my belief system. God had to remake and reshape my mind to help me discover my true identity in Him and to walk in my freedom. I had to learn to let go of my past and to forgive. Although I'm still a work in progress, I've partnered with the Holy Spirit and His word to heal and deliver me. To make me free indeed!

*Whom the Son sets free is free indeed!*

Jessica Mojica is a devoted and loving wife, a mother of four, and a grandmother to an amazing little man of God. Born and raised in Brooklyn, NY Jessica faced many challenges. Radically saved in 1998 as she grew in relationship with the Lord, Jessica discovered her true identity through the word of God. Having seen her own life transformed through the work of emotional healing, Jessica pursued and holds a Certificate of Inner Healing and Deliverance and is passionate about seeing others' lives transformed.

Jessica attends Smithtown Gospel Tabernacle where she was involved in Ancient Path Ministries helping people heal from their past. She also participates with Angel Tree Ministries where she attends people's homes to bless them with meals and gifts which her church provides during the Christmas season.

Jessica is the Founder & CEO of Prophetic Apparel 4u, with a mission to share purpose, hope, love, and to spread the gospel to a lost dying world through her clothing. Jessica is currently working on a book to help the Church deal with inner struggles, heal from their past and discover who they are in Christ.

# LEFT IN THE DARK
## MICHON WHITE BERNARD

*B*efore I share my story, I would like to establish facts that will answer some of the questions you may have. No. It was not a relative. It was a young man of a family that knew (and that at the time was somewhat close to) my family. It was not at his home. The awful incident that altered my childhood and had a long-term adverse effect on my adulthood happened inside a church. Yes, a church. Let me clarify that I lay no blame on the church, in particular the church where the incident took place. We were so close-knit; like a family. On any given Sunday afternoon, hardly anyone went home. We stayed at the church because either an afternoon or evening service would begin not too long after the morning worship service had let out. There was trust. You could leave your child in the care of just about anyone because it was like a sacred and secure village.

I can't blame the church and I can't blame the adults, especially my parents. My parents have always loved and cared for me and kept me out of harm's way. They probably would have handcuffed me to their wrists or a chair if they had known that just one moment out of their sight would be life-altering for me.

Everything was happening as it usually would. The church family was there, I was there, and other children were in what we knew as our safe place. Our church. I've often said to myself, *"Okay, if the church, my parents, other blood relatives, a host of other 'aunties' and 'uncles,' and God-fearing men and women who cared for me as their own weren't to blame, then who is to blame? Am I?"* Notice that my contemplation bent towards blaming everyone and anyone else *except* the perpetrator, which I found out later is typical for an abused victim. Somehow and in some way, I must've asked for this. I must have worn an "I'm easy" sign across my forehead. But wait, at 11, I knew nothing about *that!* So, in what way would I have given that impression? On this particular Sunday afternoon, I just existed as an 11-year-old girl named Michon.

I remember him saying, "Michon, let's go upstairs. Come on."

"Why?" I asked.

"Everyone else is up there. Come on," he answered.

At the stairs, he then took my hand in a very gentle way. It was as if he knew I was not going to scream or run. He was right. I didn't. Why was I so willing? Or was I? Maybe naive. I was eleven.

"Wait, *everyone*?! Everyone who?" I wondered. There was no service going on upstairs at the time. I should have said, "No. *Everyone* is not upstairs; you're lying!" or "Who is up there? I don't hear anyone up there." I didn't say any of that! Here I go again, self-blame. I should've said something. I should've screamed. I should've run. BUT I DIDN'T! WHY DIDN'T I?! UGH! You have no idea how many times I've persecuted myself for NOT making a move. He led me by the hand, and I just followed. Immediately, darkness hit me, but he was my guide.

I don't know if I even thought, *"something is wrong!"* No. I don't believe that I did. Instead, I trusted the hand that led me. About six to seven steps up and then another three or four. "Come here," he said. Suddenly I'm down on the steps. Now he gets a little more aggressive. I squiggle and wiggle, but the might and weight of this then sixteen or seventeen-year-old, I think, was more than I could handle. Then a forced, hard-pressed tongue kiss. A very sickening moment!

As soon as he freed my mouth, a right hand went over it, and I was told, "Shhh, it won't hurt." And as the right hand guarded my mouth, the left hand was extremely busy. The left hand worked two jobs. To unloosen his pants and then to pull down my white tights. Yes, at eleven, I was still in those. My undergarment was anxiously grabbed and then gathered by the left hand to one side. The left hand continued to work tirelessly and very quickly. The right hand then came off the mouth, and the tongue went back in. He released his right hand from its duty to assist the left. This move would be the final adjustment before he would accomplish his mission. The next moment, I remember all too well, but I will not give any more details. All I will say is painful. Oh, so awful and painful in more ways than one.

After standing to redress himself, he was courteous enough to extend his right arm and hand for me to take and lift me. His next to last words were, "You better not say anything to anybody." I didn't reply; I think shock had taken over. And then these last words, "Let me go out first." By that, he meant he would exit out of the same doors that we came in TOGETHER, by himself. Now, left alone in the dark came the real test. Did I know every square inch of this church like I thought I did? Yeah, I did. But it didn't seem like it now. I had to feel my way along the wall and proceed SLOWLY down the stairs. And then, finally. I opened the doors and stepped into the light. But for a long time, my life would still be in the dark.

At the age of 11, I did not know how to "label" my feelings. All I knew was what I felt. I remember specifically that by the age of 12, I had an overwhelming sense of "not being good enough." I then became inclined to believe that I was only good enough for the one thing, which someone took advantage of me to get. I had no idea of who my true self was, and I became promiscuous in my early teens.

When you have experienced a traumatic event such as I, the labels of insecurity, fear, rejection, and loneliness seem to self-affix. You don't need anyone to tell you what you are. You feel it. You feel the effects of what occurred. I didn't know how much the feelings would intertwine with my thoughts and how I would become or wear those thoughts or how they would grow to become long-lasting and, at times, ruthlessly overwhelming.

From 11 years old through early adulthood, through a failed first marriage, and then as a full-grown adult and single mother of two, I battled with these labels, not understanding them and not knowing that they would all merge at depression. Because I did not want to be on medication with two small children, I chose just to fight my way through, and a battle it was! There I was, in my 30's and 40's, still looking at these labels in my life and seeing the manifestation of them. I would cry out, "Lord, help me!" Indeed, He would hear me, and I would experience a great sense of relief, but it was not abiding. It would only last for a little while, and then I was back at fighting them, which wearied me to no end. I then realized that I needed counseling. It would be my first time, and I had to wrestle with whether it was the right thing to do. After all, I am saved, sanctified, and filled with the Holy Ghost. Will I "grieve" Him? Will God be mad with me? Am I opening the door to evil spirits? Do I not have faith, like I thought I did, in the power of God? How come the name of Jesus is not enough? Oh, the onslaught of questions and thoughts!

I was seeing a counselor, and then after some time, a Christian coach. Both helped; however, it was something my coach said to me that prompted a breakthrough moment. He said, "Your desire to change must be greater than your desire to remain the same." That was an epiphany moment for me because I knew I had the desire to change. And now I knew that all I needed to do was focus on being different rather than focusing on the labels that repeatedly dictated to me who I was. I will now share some critical discoveries with you as I continue to outlive my labels. Note that each one has Scripture support. I assume that you know I could not even begin to outlive my labels without God, praying for His help and His Word. He was with me all along my journey. If you have gone through the same incident or something similar, perhaps you will find that you can use these discoveries as well.

1.  The incident was not my fault, but healing was my responsibility. This discovery told me that I would have to respond to the labels with spiritual ability from within.

    *Scripture support: Ephesians 3:20 NLT - Now all glory to God, who is able, through his mighty power at work within us, to accomplish infinitely more than we might as or think.*

2.  My breakthrough was in what I feared; CHANGE. This discovery helped me see that the only way I would defeat the labels was to dare to BE different from what they dictated.

    *Scripture support: 2 Timothy 1:7 NLT - For God has not given us a spirit of fear and timidity, but of power, love, and self-discipline.*

    *2 Corinthians 5:17 NLT - This means that anyone who belongs to Christ has become a new person. THE OLD LIFE IS GONE; A NEW LIFE HAS BEGUN! (all caps mine).*

3.  I compared my labels to the label on a can that sits on the supermarket shelf. Per the FDA, the label MUST change if the ingredients change, no matter how slight the change might be. This discovery

encouraged me to give myself credit for every internal change made, whether minor or significant. It's okay for change to happen slowly as long as it is consistent. With each change, the labels are gradually peeling away, and I am outliving them.

*Scripture support: 2 Corinthians 3:18 NLT - So all of us who have had that veil removed can see and reflect the glory of the Lord. And the Lord - who is the Spirit - makes us more and more like him as we are changed into His glorious image.*

Pastor Michon White-Bernard was born in Brooklyn, New York, to Bishop J.C. and Lady Gloria White. By the time Pastor White-Bernard was in her teens, she had accepted a higher call to preach the Gospel. She attended the New England Bible Institute and began her call to Evangelism in 1988. During this time, she also served as Musician, Lead Psalmist, and Choir Director for her local church. After serving in this capacity for many years, she served as an Elder. God then called her to the Pastorate in 2001. For ten years, she was the Pastor of Lighthouse Christian Community Church in New Haven, CT. In 2010 she resigned from the Pastorate at Lighthouse to serve alongside her father, Sr. Pastor, Bishop John C. White of Cathedral of Praise C.O.G.I.C., Int'l. in Bridgeport, CT.

Pastor White-Bernard currently holds a bachelor's degree in Biblical Studies from the North Carolina College of Theology. She is a Certified Life Coach and founder of A New U, a Life Coaching company that provides individual and group, Bible-based coaching for spiritual transformation. She also specializes in Spiritual Gift Coaching. In addition to assisting the Pastorate at her church, she serves as the Director of Sanctuary Ministries and one of the Lead Praise & Worship Psalmists.

Pastor White-Bernard has graced the pulpit of many notable Pastors such as Bishop Hezekiah Walker, Pastor Donald McClurkin, and many others. She was a guest of Bishop George Bloomer on the Word Network-Rejoice in the Word television show. She is a dynamic and exceptionally gifted speaker. She uses a charismatic style of teaching, stressing spiritual transformation, and growth. She is fully committed to the believer's total growth and development in every phase, both naturally and spiritually. She is committed to the biblical principles that build the Body of Christ.

# BETTER OFF DEAD
## DORIS BROWN

*I*n our lifetime we experience things that cause twist and turns. Well, my life experience started in my mother's womb. She had no idea that I was even conceived, which is sometimes called a mistake or unplanned conception. I was the one that God had chosen to cross the threshold into this expedition. On September 14, 1967, her bundle of joy arrived. Anticipating the arrival of her chucky buttercup infant, she lovingly expected her unborn to come into the world perfect. This was not so; her newborn was born with a defect. It was noticed that she had a club foot. After placing a cast on the infant, the long-term mobility issues began. After years of wearing special shoes to prevent the foot from twisting back, I was dead set on walking straight and upright, not realizing that naturally it was thought provoking clips of what I must do spiritually. In other words, life will serve you issues. It will always want you to turn back. But taking preventive actions is in order. What I was born with, I no longer gave it the go-ahead to survive. Now I have gained the power over my life in that area.

You see, I came into the world with a challenge. I had no inclination that I was going to war with the spirit of sickness and that I would ride emotional roller coasters. In the state of innocence, I was being developed and evolving into the unknown territories of what I thought life was. Battling with thoughts of, *"I'm a mistake"* I wasn't looking for understanding, but validation.

On this journey, I discovered that my life was being misguided by my flesh. There were so many conflicts and I was laboring under delusions. The pursuit of my flesh was driving into kingship while at the same time offering false hope. The more that I was engulfed with thoughts of being a mistake, my self-esteem decreased drastically. There I was thinking being in Christ would surely be a piece of my favorite cake. But that was the flesh talking and not the spirit man. Being in Christ gives you the power to go through. Comparing your life with the Word of God is the compass that will navigate you in the right direction. So, how can I keep on forgetting the very thing that's needed to get me through. This tormenting spirit misled my mind into a spiral of defeat. But I knew that I needed to gain territory – it was time to face this head on. I began to read 2 Corinthians 10:4-5, "*The weapons we fight with are not the weapons of the world. On the contrary, they have divine power to demolish strongholds. We demolish arguments and every pretension (a claim) that sets itself up against the knowledge of God, and we take captive every thought to make it obedient to Christ.*" The more I read the verses aloud, the more they came alive.

When you're ready to make your final decision to stand up for Christ specific issues will arise, designed to sculpt the clay that you are. Year after year there were so many blows, trying to remove my anchor. But each one was different and life threatening. What could I do? How could I make it through? It was like being in a boxing ring and the other opponent knew my weakness. There I was overwhelmed, panting and out of breath. The sweat, tears, and mental stress caused me to have meditations on surrendering. Now I was wounded, the pain was unbearable. Once again, I was being tortured. Quoting the Word of God is nothing like living it. I rushed to the Word of God as I struggled to stand. What did I find that overthrew those troubles? Psalm 34:19 says, *"Many are the afflictions (something that causes pain or suffering) of the righteous: but the LORD delivereth (carry out, carry through) him out of them all."* Wow, the LORD delivereth, us out of our innumerable (too many to be counted) troubles!

I immediately painted a beautiful illustration of rich green fragrant cut grass. As I was being led by the spirit of God by the still water. Though the water was inviting and calm. He made me lie down to rest. He ministered to my spirit man. As I was enclosed in His presence, all the troubles were driven away, yet still present. Simply meaning I have the ability to go through. When you are focused on fulfilling your assignment and not your flesh, you can succeed in all things.

I suffered many of what I thought were setbacks. But in all reality, they were full-fledged divine arrangements to maturity. I endured various insults, one specifically cutting to the core. I was told, "those that were sickly were better off dead and that there was no purpose for life." Instantly, questions were invading my mind such as: How can this person say this and where is their compassion? Therefore, the statement drove me to believe that I was better off dead. But I made the decision to change the verdict that was spoken over me. Choosing to be dead indeed unto sin, but alive unto God in Christ Jesus (Romans 6:11). Responding to the statement was not needed.

I'll say it was the best decision I have ever made. When you learn that you have an option, choose death. It allows you to block out the noise of distraction and helps you to focus on what is ahead. You are only subject to the spirit of GOD. You don't have to be the dumpster for everyone's opinions. Regardless of sickness, test, and trials, life after death is more rewarding. When you allow yourself to die unto the flesh, GOD will allow countless doors to be opened in your favor.

## Activity

1. Choose at least three healing and faith scriptures to continually feed your mind and memorize them.

   _____

   _____

   _____

   _____

   _____

   _____

   _____

   _____

2. Build your self-awareness by examining and journaling your emotions, thoughts, response, and your verbalizations. Also write what it should be if it goes contrary to the Word of God. Always align yourself with the Word of God. Ask God for strategies for each situation.

3. Memorize: 2 Corinthians 10:4-5; For the weapons of our warfare are not carnal, but mighty through

God to the pulling down of strongholds; Casting down imaginations, and every high thing that exalteth itself against the knowledge of God, and bringing into captivity every thought to the obedience of Christ.

4. Journal your success stories.

Apostle Doris Brown is the Founder and Senior Leader of Walk in Righteous Living Ministries in Waterbury CT. Her apostolic lifestyle demonstrates her love in rearing leaders to fulfill their God-given assignment. Apostle's love for souls is genuine, she endeavors to win and teach many for Christ so that God might be Glorified! Her aim is to consistently live victoriously in the presence of God as she steadfastly holds to the Word of the Lord.

Her motto is: But none of these things move me, neither count I my life dear unto myself, so that I might finish my course with joy, and the ministry, which I have received of the Lord Jesus, to testify the gospel of the grace of God. Acts 20:24

# PEACE AFTER UNDERSTANDING
## NORJA CUNNINGHAM, PHD, LMFT

*I*n 2009, as a part of my doctoral student experience, I started teaching masters level courses. Retrospectively, I believe my professors chose to provide opportunities for me to teach subjects where I could develop personally and professionally. I entered the program focused on my identity as a follower of Christ and did not know my beliefs would be challenged. The course focused on multiculturalism, specifically how a marriage and family therapist can respectfully provide treatment to an individual and family of a different race/ethnicity, gender, class, ability, religion/spirituality and sexual orientation. If you are a Christian and grew up in a Christian community, you know I had to challenge my narrative about these topics.

Please understand, I was raised with an awareness of my multicultural background. My Black mother was raised in a predominantly Caucasian community in Westchester County, New York. On the other hand, my Black father was raised in a rural predominantly Black town in Gordo,

Alabama and they raised me in an urban city in Connecticut. I have interracial/ interethnic couples in my family. There are LGBTQIA members in my family too. Most of my family is Christian. So, as I prepared to teach this diversity course, I thought about my family's diversity and my experience as an inner-city Black Christian female.

There were battling narratives (between the university's meaning of multiculturalism and my belief system) in my mind. I had to be honest about my biases, check my biases and still remain authentic to my beliefs. I wondered, how am I going to challenge this all white class to think about diversity? I knew I could effortlessly teach them about my ethnic and racial differences. But how were they going to appreciate the diversity that was not as clear among their whiteness? I was a bit nervous when I knew the classes were approaching the discussions about religion and sexual orientation. Why? I was attending a university that valued social justice. The state motto is "Live Free or Die" and I thought of Harriet Tubman when I learned this. I was living in a town that raised rainbow and confederate flags; owls, half-moons and stars were everywhere (signifying wicca). According to a Gallup poll, 20% of New Hampshire residents reported being "very religious" and became known as the least religious state in the U.S. (2016). Therefore, I didn't know if the very religious were in my class or not. I wondered how they would respond to me as their professor, and how they would respond to the discussion topics. I also wondered if I was going to be accepted, as I knew I was not fully accepted since day one because of being Christian. Then I had to acknowledge my biases regarding race/ethnicity, religion, class, ability, gender and sexual orientation to honor every student attending my class. I found myself going through this psychological process as I prepared for every class and I made it through the entire semester — all 16 weeks! Thank God! The students reported they learned a lot and appreciated my ability to remain mostly unbiased and be an example of openly acknowledging my biases in a respectful manner.

The multicultural course challenged me to dig deep and truly learn to live the scripture, "God is love" (1 John 4:16) and the first scripture I learned as a youth (John 3:16), "For God so loved the world..." When I say that I mean, I learned I am not responsible for judging my students, and so I released myself from that expectation. That action made me aware of how, some of us Christians are socialized to be judgmental. We can be judgmental without awareness of it. Ultimately, judgment is up to God, according to Romans 2:6-8. In other words, God owns heaven and hell. I do not determine who goes where. Therefore, it is not my burden to judge anyone or I will be judged as harshly as I judged them (Matthew 7:1-2). We have free will to decide how we will live our lives (Deuteronomy 30:15). Ultimately, I was able to love each student as he/she/they presented him/her/themselves in my class. That diversity course taught me to be a better Christian.

Conclusively, I had students engaging in respectful conversation with me and each other — who were white, openly straight, gay, lesbian, bisexual, transgender, wiccan, atheist, satanist, agnostic, feminist, suffering with a disability, from blue collar families or white-collar families or any combination of what was listed. I was also able to learn how to meditate. I saw this experience as my first triumph during my doctoral studies. I started the program as the Christian Black Heterosexual female who they thought was homophobic and closed-minded. While teaching, I became the Christian Black Heterosexual woman from an urban city who was different than their usual encounters. I was able to outlive the label of being perceived as a prejudice Christian.

With God as the source of my strength, I accomplished much during my doctoral education and after graduating. My Vietnamese American female and Turkish Muslim female cohort colleagues, friends, sisters and I completed a qualitative research study that highlighted the phenomenon of immigration for three generations. This study turned into an international presentation at an IFTA (International Family Therapy Association) Conference hosted in Argentina. I completed my dissertation, graduated from the doctoral program in August 2015 and since that time, I've met every Christian Black woman who attended the same institution. I was able to supervise, teach or extend my support during their doctoral process. In some ways, I felt a deeper connection to the "Live Free or Die" motto like Harriet Tubman viewed it. I was able to see others through the wilderness of the PWI (predominantly white institution) doctoral experience and witness them receive their doctoral degrees. Now, I am currently active on the dissertation committee of the first Christian African male who will be graduating from the same program I and the three other Christian Black women finished. All of these accomplishments made all of my cultural clashes and understandings worth the battles. We earned our degrees and respect. We are winning. I represent a great group of thriving educated Christian Black people. Thankfully, I am not the only one. I just happened to be the first who graduated from my doctoral program. It is our time. Let's keep winning, as we crush those labels!

## Lessons

1. Sometimes, people need time to get to know you to refute their biases and stereotypes about your culture. Then, being different can be an asset to the relationship.

2. It is possible to be an intellectual, learn about other cultures, and still follow Jesus Christ.

3. The challenging of your faith teaches you where you are strong in your faith and where more work on your faith is required.

4. New experiences expand your cultural capacity and maintaining your spiritual foundation is your responsibility.

5. When you know who you are, others cannot influence you to engage in ungodly behavior.

# REFERENCES

Gallup (February 4, 2016). "New Hampshire Now Least Religious State in U.S." Gallup.com. Retrieved December 23, 2020.

Inspired by God (2007). King James Version, Life applications study bible. Carol Stream, IL: Tyndale House Publishers, Inc.

Dr. Cunningham received her Bachelor of Science in psychology from Trinity College, her Master of Science in Marriage and Family Therapy from Central Connecticut State University, and her doctoral degree in marriage and family therapy from Antioch University New England. Her undergraduate research focused on the impact of media on the body image and self-esteem of Black females in early adulthood. Her doctoral dissertation was a phenomenological study focused on how compassion fatigue in therapists can affect their marriages and families.

Dr. Cunningham is a licensed marriage and family therapist, who has been providing clinical treatment to individuals, families and couples through her private practice since January 2015. In total, Dr. Cunningham has been providing mental health services to individuals, couples and families since 2005. She specializes in trauma, grief and relational therapy. In line with her specialties, she is trained in Trauma-Focused Cognitive Behavioral Therapy, Accelerated Resolution Therapy (ART) and is a certified facilitator of the Prepare-Enrich program.

Most recently, Dr. Cunningham has published *#LifeLessons: Facebook Wisdom*, *#LifeLessons: FB Wisdom Revamped Workbook* and *#LifeLessons: A Workbook for Grieving Children (& Parents)* —available on Amazon. All of her information can be found on her website www.necllc.website, her Facebook page NEC, and her Instagram page @neclmft.

# NEVER WAS ENOUGH
## ALEXIS NICOLE

"Never" should've been my middle name. Growing up as a misfit in a socially impaired world gave me only one option and that was to fail. Sometimes I blame my mother for the way life treated me. No preparation, no guidance; just a pat on the back and I'll see you after work was all I got. The stigma and pressure of being a strong black woman was the label my momma was given and for that, it will always have a negative imprint in my heart.

"Never" followed me from birth. My mother *never* married my father. She *never* wanted kids and I *never* felt the true impact of love from either of my parents. As a kid I *never* fit in at school because I was academically above average in a poverty stricken remedial inner-city school district. My peers grew up in the projects while I lived in a one family home. They used to get free lunch while I had a stupid Barbie lunch box. They rode on the school bus while my great-aunt used to pick me up with "Lady" our old Collie dog. Riding in a 1990 Ford Taurus station wagon automatically put me in the "Offie" category, and it also didn't help that I was overweight. The label of fighting to fit in followed me for the next 20-plus years of my life.

Looking back if I were to pinpoint the exact moment where I first began to dance with the devil, I would have to say it was summers at my great aunt's cottage. I was so excited my cousins were coming to stay for a few weeks. Finally, someone to play with, hang out and stay up all night with. It wasn't too long before "never" crept in and followed me to the bottom bunk of my fire engine red full-size bunkbed. My mom never knew when I broke my virginity. How could I tell her I was having sex with my older cousin? Well, my justification at 11 years old was that we were only family by marriage, so this couldn't be so bad; or so I thought. Every time he wanted to play these strange games, I never said no. Molestation only happens when you say "NO" right? Later on, I realized that my abandonment issues from my parents caused me to leave an "open door policy" for men, and even at one-point women that walked into my life.

Summer of '95 was over and finally I was going to middle school. Everything about me had changed. My demeanor, my attitude, and even worse my sexuality. Sexually, I was never ready for what was going to happen to me and funny thing is life didn't care! My cousin (now in high school) was a few blocks away. I figured I'd skip school and go see him. Maybe he missed me; my kitty sure did. As I approached the school in efforts to try and find him everything in me said "turn around." I found him on the breezeway on the upper westside hallway of the school. I ran up to him so excited in hopes that he would be happy to see me.

My excitement quickly flickered away as I approached his mortified face which was covered with disgust. He looked me up and down and then said, "What the hell are you doing here?" Surprised by his response, I grabbed him by the hand and batted my eyes like I was a damsel in distress. Maybe he didn't recognize me? Puberty did hit me in all the right places by that time. He snatched his hand away and told me to leave and dismissed me by walking away. Standing there a strong black cloud shaded over me and I knew from that moment, I was not going to see him again; so, I put every effort in trying to replace him with any Tom, Dick or Harry.

As the years passed my attempts to find a replacement sizzled and failed. Desperate times called for desperate measures and I found myself in a downward spiral of dysfunctional toxic relationships for the next twenty years. It didn't matter if it was a man, woman, old or young; nothing ever panned out. I never thought God had a plan for my life. I didn't know who "God" was. My life was all about fast money, drugs and sex. Whatever Lexy wanted; Lexy got! Never, ever could I fathom my New Year's 2013 experience. While I was supposed to be sitting in a church pew, I decided to switch destinations and things drastically took a turn for the worse.

Bottle after bottle, pill after pill, blunt after blunt; never could I have expected that right before I blacked out that over five men would brutally rape me. Waking up naked in an empty room with only tiny horrific flashbacks of the night before, I finally concluded that if there was a God He needed to intervene now. Understanding that Jezebel had become my alter ego, I knew soon she was going to consume me if I didn't find a way out. Proverbs 23:28 says, "She lurks *and* lies in wait like a robber [who waits for prey], And she increases the faithless among men."

After all that I survived, rape victim was the only label that I could not overcome. Raped? How could I ever be set free from that? Shoot, domestic violence could not even hold me bound! I set my mind a long time ago to believe that the next negro who decided to put his hands on me was gonna meet his maker, if my fist could not fix him! So, what was it about my sexuality that kept me captive? As I reflect on the healing process that it took to overcome what I experienced in my life, I can honestly say that God is the only thing that healed me. As an emotional creature, a daughter, a woman and most importantly a mother, there are so many layers to how we connect and how we react to things. God did not design us to "just get over it." It's not that simple. The beauty beyond the mask has an opportunity to replenish itself and that flower must be watered once it withers. Yes, watered by the word of God and the Holy Spirit.

Deliverance is what has helped me to go from victim to survivor, promiscuous woman to wife, and drug addict to minister. The labels that the world convicted me by have no power or prosperity over God's plan. However, surrendering my life over to God was a part of the process. The other part was therapy. Just as long as it took to create my problems, it now takes even more consistent time to undo what was done. It's a shame how the stigma of going to see a "therapist" deems you as crazy yet the ones who DON'T go to see one are the same people who act the WORST! Talking about it, crying to get a release, and getting that junk off my chest revived my heart and restored my love for self. My past is behind me and my future looks too bright to ever allow my pain to dictate where I am going.

Minister Alexis Nicole is a wife with a blended family of five children, the CEO of Holy Drip Cosmetics LLC, a licensed minister, and a full-time student at Liberty University with a major in Biblical and Theological Studies. She has overcome many obstacles in her life like becoming a teenage mother, domestic violence, rape, drug addiction and even incarceration. However, Alexis is a survivor and her passion for advocating for women with trauma is a priority to her. She is currently writing her debut novel and inspirational guide about learning how to overcome the "dry" areas in your life. As a 2017 graduate of the Black Ministries program at the Hartford Seminary, she wants the world to know you can do anything you put your mind to. Step out of the box and live; ANYTHING IS POSSIBLE!!! "They thought I'd be a statistic and nothing but a hood chick living in the ghetto...but look at me now. I'm out here breaking barriers and showing people there is life after abuse. Becoming a survivor is only the beginning!"

# THE THREE R'S OF BECOMING:
## REGRET, RECALIBRATE, AND RELEASE
### YVONNE BOWEN

*"Trauma is the most avoided, ignored, belittled, denied, misunderstood, and untreated cause of human suffering."*
— Peter Levine

*"If you don't get out there and define yourself, you'll be quickly and inaccurately defined by others."*
— Michelle Obama

*"As I walked out the door toward the gate that would lead to my freedom, I knew if I didn't leave my bitterness behind, I'd still be in prison."*
— Nelson Mandela

**Regret**

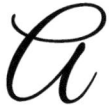 s a young woman then in her 20s excited about working one of her first real jobs out of high school I would carpool into work with my Dad. I

was so nervous about doing a good job, and worried about making my Dad proud of me taking steps to become a responsible young woman in society. The lesson of office politics mixed with sexual favors was the last thing I thought I would learn about when I took the job, but it quickly became par for the course as an African American woman working in corporate White America. As my days were measured by avoiding passes, being groped and hearing off-color sexual remarks in a tight file room daily, 5:00pm could never arrive soon enough each day. What I tried to ignore soon could not be ignored by my shy younger self who had not found her voice yet but knew that this was wrong.

## Recalibrate

Having put my trust in the leadership of the office, who had never given me any other reason to believe that there would be an issue if I brought a problem to him, I reported the harassments to the department manager. Much to my surprise and disappointment, after sharing that both of my co-workers were repeatedly brushing up against me and making inappropriate sexual comments despite my repeated requests to stop, I was accused of leading them on and then fired. How could this be? I followed the rules! Why was I the victim being treated like the one who did something wrong?

The confusion and cognitive dissonance that followed made for the perfect antagonists for bitterness, anger, hyper-sensitivity, unforgiveness and shame. The whirlwind of fear, shame, doubt and victimization became common themes I had to overcome, but how? Raised in a suburban spiritual family the tools to deal with this kind of injustice just were not there. While I knew they loved me and cared about me, I was blessed if they could at least listen to me vent. How to overcome it all would be lessons and tools that later God would instill later in my life. *Integrated Listening* defines trauma as the response to a deeply distressing or disturbing event that overwhelms an individual's ability to cope, causes feelings of helplessness, and diminishes their sense of self and their ability to feel a full range of emotions and experiences.[1] In the moment I heard the words *"You're fired!"*, I was crushed. The clear retaliation for telling the truth, rocked my core. Becoming who you are to be in life is a quest that is full of stops and starts, but the trick is often to start again after the worst stops that are usually the result of trauma. While I have learned many years later that some of the wisest words uttered after an experience like this is *"Let's begin again."* But that was the last thing I wanted to do! There was a deep sense of despair, depression and even shame. One of the lessons I learned was just how powerful the mind is depending on how you are thought to think or process a thing; it can make all the difference in mere survival or overcoming and thriving a thing.

Studies show that when we are forced in a furnace of a traumatic episode in life and emotionally or mentally ruminate over an experience, we become indoctrinated in a proverbial programming loop and negativity effects our

---

[1]  13, February 2021. "What Is Trauma? - Definition, Symptoms, Responses, Types & Therapy." Integrated Listening, Integrated Listening, 28 Jan. 2021, < integratedlistening.com/what-is-trauma/>.

bodies even down to the cellular level. So much so it is like putting yourself on a toxic medical IV drip of biochemical neurotransmitters creating your physical reality[2]. In other words, what we think can manifest in disease, headaches, aliments, etc. The body is all interconnected and when bad information is not processed out mentally, it will manifest physically in the body through cellular disease, rashes or other disorders.[3] Research shows that about 87% of illness can be attributed to our thought life whereas only diet, genetics and environment only account for 13%.[4] Our bodies have memory and when we do not deal with the toxicity of a situation, place, or thing it will hold on to the bad information until we make peace of it.

Trauma does not discriminate, and it is pervasive throughout the world. A World Mental Health survey conducted by the World Health Organization found that at least a third of the more than 125,000 people surveyed in 26 different countries had experienced trauma. That number rose to 70% when the group was limited to people experiencing core disorders as defined by the DSM-IV (the classification found in the *Diagnostic and Statistical Manual of Mental Disorders, 4th Edition*). But those numbers are just for instances that have been reported; the actual number is

---

[2] Leaf, Dr. Caroline. *Who Switched Off My Brain? Controlling Toxic Thoughts and Emotions.* Dallas, Texas: Switch on Your Brain USA, Inc., 2008.

[3] Colbert, Dr. Don. Deadly Emotions: Understanding the Mind-Body-Spirit Connection that can Heal or Destroy You. Nashville Texas: Thomas Nelson Publishing, May 2006.

[4] Leaf, 2008.

probably, much higher.[5] Science has made direct correlations between emotional trauma such as anxiety, stress as a result of prolonged depression, increased risk for heart disease, cancer, heart angina/palpitation, arthritis and more.[6] Time is a precious commodity and due to Covid-19 we have more time to ponder and process the motives, missteps of others and ourselves in a more meaningful way. You can literally assist your body in healing by thinking your way to a healthier you. As Orval Hobart Mowrer, the originator of the phrase said, and echoes scripture (Luke 12:2, NIV) "we are as sick as our secrets." It is through our courage to deal with what happened do we find life.

**Release it!**

I challenge you to do the following to process through your pain to be powerful and fully present in life again:

1.  Find a quiet space away from the new distractions of this pandemic bubble we live in and allow yourself to be ministered to by the Holy Spirit to bring back to your memory the incidents that you have buried from your past but still have not dealt with.

2.  Write down whatever feelings come to mind and

---

[5]  13, February 2021. "What Is Trauma? - Definition, Symptoms, Responses, Types & Therapy." *Integrated Listening*, Integrated Listening, 28 Jan. 2021, < integratedlistening.com/what-is-trauma/>.

[6]  Leaf, Dr. Caroline. Who Switched Off My Brain? Controlling Toxic Thoughts and Emotions. Dallas, Texas: Switch off Your Brain USA, Inc., 2008.

the incident(s). Write any "isms" or behavioral changes after the incident. Identification of change is key to start the journey to your best you. Then allow yourself if you have not already, to begin to feel the pain again while allowing yourself to process the why behind it and record it. Do not run from the pain of the incident! Do embrace it to heal.

3. Then confess, "I forgive myself and the person who hurt me. I am safe now; it is over, and we are okay." The "we" here is you then and you are now. Take three deep breaths. Allow yourself to be fully aware to every bit of that experience and then let it go and exhale.

4. Now write down how you feel after releasing the pain of the situation and intaking the newness of thought that you are well, and you are safe now.

5. This last step will be a reoccurring one that you can modify however you desire. Now find two people who know you the best but are not enablers of any negative isms you may have but will tell you the truth in love. Make sure that these are not people who will not weaponize what you share but will honor what you share to help you grow past your trauma. Ask them how you treat others, and what they have observed about you good and bad since the time of the incident(s). It is not most important that they know what happened, but rather that they

are a loving objective barometer. If you do not feel comfortable talking with them about it just ask them to write it and then repeat the steps.

The journey from trauma to triumph is one that begins with continual steps of courage one step at a time. Not every step or decision will work out perfectly. Do not expect it to but be gentle with yourself and allow yourself to deal with the process, the pivotal moments and unique people in your life. Allow yourself to recover and release it so you can recalibrate yourself to who God truly intended for you to be. Throw away the regrets, the shame and start anew one step, one day at a time and one crisis at a time. You've got this!

Yvonne Bowen is a prophetic worship artist. She is a certified Liturgical Dance Teacher. She is the proud mother of one son and grandmother of two beautiful grandchildren; she currently resides in Danielson, CT.

Her relationship with the Lord started at the early the age of 13. She has been dancing for the Lord since 2003 working with various churches to grow their Dance Ministries, preaching, teaching, and working in the vineyard for over 28 years. She has been a member of the National Liturgical Dance Network via its CT Chapter since 2007. She has faithful served as a Dance Minister is the Founder of Steps to Victory.

Her education and background include training in Prophetic Movement, Liturgical Dance Education, Small Business Management, a Baccalaureate Degree in Individualized Studies from Charter Oak College in New Britain, CT, a Graduate Certificate in Ministry in Daily Life from Hartford Seminary in Hartford, CT. She is also a graduate of the Black Ministries Program and Women's Leadership Institute of Hartford Seminary.

# TRAUMA & TRIGGERS YET TRIUMPHANT
## JOLI BLOUNT

*a*s I write this I recount the past 10 months where we have been living through one of the worst pandemics we have had in over more than a century. The current number of those impacted is traumatizing. We have a total of 22,000,000 COVID-19 cases, with an increase of 225,000 new cases, 4,000 plus deaths daily and a death toll of over 360,000 people. Every home has been impacted in some form or another whether a loss of a loved one, a close friend, a job or even infection. Thankfully help is on the horizon as the federal government has approved multiple vaccines with a 94% proof of being effective. The economy has taken a global shift as individuals has experienced such deep caves in perpetual darkness searching for moments of recovery from this globe pandemic trauma. No one could have ever made sense of this. I, too, experience battling a COVID-19 case in the spring of 2020. The recovery of trauma for me was that of something similar to the trauma I'd experienced and wrote about it in *Outlive the Labels Volume I* chapter titled, *Public Pain Privately Rewarded.* In Volume I, I elaborated the depth of affliction I'd experienced and its consequence of action after being labeled for years based on a misguided act.

First, let's take a moment to look at the word trauma. Trauma in the English language is a word that has a duality of meaning. The word trauma is often used biblically as the word "wound." In the Greek language the etymology of the word originated from the Greek word *titrosko* meaning "to wound." Luke, the great physician, referenced it in Luke 10:34 in his teaching about the Parable of the Good Samaritan. He spoke of the Good Samaritan bounding up an injured persons wounds, pouring in oil and wine, then setting him on his own beast, bringing him to an inn, and taking care of him. Similar to that in which a hospital describes trauma. In the hospital its relative to that of the severity and meaning of an injury.

The word trauma may also be used at the scene of a crime when the police are assessing someone assaulted or perhaps when dealing with a degree of head trauma occurring from a hammer, an axe, or even some type of brutal beating. The type of savage crime that it is almost unimaginable. Generally, this type of trauma is referenced as medically related. Psychologists also use the word trauma, but it has a different inference. A psychologist may deem trauma as psychological. This type of trauma damages a person's mind as a result of one or more distressing events causing overwhelming amounts of stress that exceed the person's ability to cope or integrate the emotions involved, eventually leading to serious, long-term negative consequences. I personally experienced moments of extreme psychological anguish by being labeled dumb, stupid, whore and worthless. Each moment and experience of labeling created an anxiety for me. Mentally I felted shamed, betrayed , and rejected and not just within the context of relationships. Yet in job opportunities, both in my local church and community, I often felt oppressed and isolated with no way out.

When experiencing these types of emotional events, it threatens ones very sense of safety, the absence of good things, or the presence of bad things within the context of relationships; a person's whole being is impacted — body, spirit, mind, and soul. Everyone has experienced trauma at some level in ways that have influenced our belief systems, emotions, and responses to God and others. Negative emotions or affliction is not something human beings enjoy. Our human nature is to seek pleasure and avoid pain. We especially do not revel in being put down, persecuted, oppressed, rejected, or abused. Anything that happens to us, or something we witness that is unpredictable, out of our control, and threatens our sense of safety or the safety of those we love can be defined as a trauma.

*Has it ever occurred to you that Jesus experienced trauma?*

In the first few years of Jesus' life, Jesus' parents were forced to move to Egypt because the ruler at the time was ordering that all baby boys be killed. Here, their sense of safety was certainly threatened. Once he began living out His calling, His cousin John the Baptist, whom prepared the way for Him, was beheaded. Jesus was betrayed in the garden and unjustly accused of crimes that He knew would lead to His death. Traumatically beaten and bruised, His very own community rejected Him and saved a ruthless criminal's life instead. Jesus suffered the experience of death on a cross; the death of a criminal in agony and shame.

I would like for you to take a moment and think of a time when you were in a fight physically and/or mentally. How traumatic was this event for you? If it's too traumatic for you to unpack in this setting I would recommend speaking with a professional to help you unpack it in a healthy way as this moment may trigger some emotion you're not sure how to handle on your own. If you are able to unpack it on your own, remind yourself of how you overcame it. Often times the win is simply in you serving the trauma. You're still here so let's celebrate that fact that you are triumphant. You should celebrate each time you have overcome or served something. Even God celebrated each day after creating the earth. In Genesis after each day He would exclaim, "It is good!"

There is a process that leads to the promise, and in the process, you have to take baby steps and learn how to celebrate yourself. Draw into your life a reflection of yourself. We are in a perpetual state of trauma often causing triggers, however we don't take advantage of the triumphant. As Bishop T.D. Jakes once stated, the trauma may last for a period of time; however, did you seek overcoming it by celebrating just as long? Triumphant is sometimes just being here. In other words, you made it! The devil tried to take me out yet I'm still here.

Afflictions are a part of life. It's not what happens to us but largely our responsibility on what we do with what happen to us. I chose to make these afflictions profitable; maximizing every opportunity to glorify God. If you're experiencing some form of affliction know that you will overcome it and win in the end.

Transform your PTSD to
Powerful Purpose
P. T .S. D.
*Past. Traumas. Stressors. Dis-ease*

Posture your pain to prosper in your purpose

Turn your Trauma and Triggers into Triumph

Starve your Stressors and focus on your Savior

Ditch your Dis-ease and dash to your Destiny

Joli Blount is an accomplished businesswoman, entrepreneur, best-selling author, speaker, philanthropist, mentor, coach and a licensed minister at The Potter's House of Dallas. She is the founder and CEO of Mirroring Image, LLC where she provides business consulting and project management services & Impact for Community Change a 501 (c) (3) non-profit organization where IFCC serves as an advocate for building stronger communities globally. As the first of her siblings to attend college and graduate with a Master's in Business Administration with a concentration in Project Management her passion waxed strong in her desire to cultivate a community that would reflect her dream. This illuminated her interest in education, economic empowerment, and leadership. She is a staunch believer that aptitude is universal, however opportunity is not.

When she is not pursing her career endeavors in business management and the non-profit sector, Joli enjoys preaching, teaching, and exhortation as she helps her 30-plus University Student partners become the best version of self through self-efficacy, community engagement and volunteerism. She takes pleasure in traveling, cooking, spending time with her son, working-out, reading, listening to music, hosting events, fashion, movies, and volunteering in the community and at her church.

# FROM THE PIT TO THE PALACE
## FLORENCE MARSHALL

*O*n July 21, 1985 a future mover and shaker by the name of Florence Lillian Marshall entered into the world without a care or worry. Not knowing years of her life would include abandonment, suffering, tests and trials, being misunderstood, and thoughts of feeling like Christ himself *"Why has thou forsaken me."* See, on July 21st while my mother was pushing me out, my natural father abandoned my mother and I without a care. My mother instantly went into survival mode as she began the process of motherhood without a manual. One thing I can say is she relied on Jesus, and with His favor she encamped a major Christ-filled village around us to raise me up in the things of God.

Although my mom went through her season of not having much, she did the best she could. She made sure I had food, clothes, and shelter — we came out alright. My mom let me know how the pain of being on welfare was because she didn't like to depend on anyone to assist her and felt helpless. God used my anointed Godparents, the late A.

Joel and Beatrice Somerville, along with my adopted Grandparents, Archbishop J.C. White and his loving wife Gloria, to assist my mother along with a few others in raising me in the admonition of the lord.

I am a young lady whose journey began at the age of five — being told I would be in Special Education. My grandfather anointed me and instructed my mother to have me take their test and evaluation. The evaluators were stunned! I not only outscored their test, but also their evaluation in the city and State of Connecticut. The teacher that tried to put me in Special Education confessed and said she didn't know what to do with a gifted student like me since I loved to sing so much. I was then told in the sixth grade by my teacher that I wouldn't amount to-anything. I was told I would only achieve a middle school diploma. Here I am today a young lady that graduated with honors from high school, earned 15 college credits, received one of the most prestigious State of Connecticut awards for the overall graduating class of 2003, went on to earn my Associates, Bachelors, Double Masters, Graduate Women's Studies Certificate, and a post-master's in educational leadership, to currently working on my Doctoral dissertation!

Throughout my journey I was teased, put down, laughed, and mocked for being poor, different, rejected, called, and anointed by God. In elementary and middle school, I was told I would lay on my back, have over eight kids, and would live in poverty all my life! Yet, here I am today letting you know I've outlived the labels. Yes, I came from poverty. No, I didn't have much, but now I have a full-time job working on my journey to be the CEO of the

Kingdom City Academy for Music and Arts. I have two life insurance policies, I live in two states, and I had the honor of ministering the Gospel through Word and song on local, state, national, and international levels.

I'll never forget the day when I auditioned for a major choir I wanted to be a part of and was told "No, you don't have what it takes to be a part of us from the money, sound, look, and more." My heart was broken, wounded, battered because I looked up to this particular choir. There were Sundays when I would have to sit in the pew when this choir sang, yet broken because I wanted to belong. Approximately eight years later the Lord allowed major doors to open up for me to sing for major national gospel recording artists through G.M.W.A. (Gospel Music Workshop of America), COGIC (National Church of God in Christ) as a front-line singer, and with Pastor Vincent Bohanan and the Sound of Victory where I began singing internationally. I thought my pain was over, but it wasn't. People would secretly ask me who I slept with to get to the top and say mean things like *"you're here, you're there, you're everywhere"* not knowing that was a major insult to my heart.

What I am thankful for is even in the midst of the great poverty, depression, and oppression that my mother and I had to endure, we made it out. I'll never forget the love of Mother Willie Coverson, who made sure anytime I came to her house I always had something to eat, take showers if needed, or just be right there for me to talk to in my time of need. As the time grew my mother met and married my step-father, the late Mr. Ora Vines, who provided a permanent house for us in Bridgeport, Connecticut. Even in the midst of that we overcame hard times within our home. From no heat and hot water to our family being separated for almost 15 years, God brought us back as a family before my late step-father passed in August of 2020. In the midst of us healing as a family, and my step-father making it through his last days on earth we were blessed with my niece Robyn Renee who is our gift from God as my dad now rests on in God. Truly she brought us a beacon of hope!

After all I endured, I became the first African-American woman at Western Connecticut State University to be inducted into Iota Iota Iota (National Women's Studies Honor Society) and served on various state and national leadership roles. I was blessed to attend Fordham University and graduate. My former Dean told me to give it up because I didn't have the money to continue... ha! The Lord not only gave me a major scholarship to finish my program, but I end up graduating with extended funding, Presidential recognition, a Fordham elite, and more!

I went from having nothing to now grateful for all that God has done and getting ready to do!-I'm grateful that God didn't allow the naysayers and the doubters to have their way in my life! Truly, my story is: "From the Pit to the Palace — I'm not where you left me!"

Min. Florence Lillian Marshall was born on July 21, 1985 to Missionary Ruth Vines and Gary Wallace in Bridgeport, CT. Florence was educated in the Bridgeport Public School

System and have been tremendously blessed to have earned various degrees from Housatonic Community College, Western Connecticut State, Fordham University, and currently Capella University as she is currently pursuing her doctoral in Educational Leadership and Management. Florence accepted the Lord Jesus Christ and received the gift of the Holy Spirit at an early age. Florence serves at Cathedral of Praise Church of God in Christ, where her adopted Grandparents Arch-Bishop Elect J.C. White and Evangelist Gloria White serve as the pastors. Florence serves as a minister, national adjutant, and a psalmist. She serves the church on local, national, and international levels. Beyond all that she is a servant! Flo's motto: "Impacting one's life for Christ one day at a time."

# SHE FIGHTS
## D. MICHELLE BENNETT

his is the story of a fighter who grew up with loving parents, but a toxic village. There was never a shortage of love, however, at times I felt isolated. I had all brothers and living in a house full of men, there was no room for the softness of a girl. So, I learned to be tough. My home was loving but I always sought acceptance from my village. I wanted to belong, but I was never able to fit. My village rejected me, and I carried that rejection which affected my ability to form lasting friendships, relationships, and meaningful connections. I was a broken little girl who longed to be accepted and loved; so much so that I ended up in relationships and situations that further damaged an already scarred soul trying to find that acceptance and validation. I ended up sacrificing a lot of who I was to keep people around.

I admit I was rough around the edges. I had a relentless attitude and sharp tongue, but I developed that tough image to protect an already fragile heart after repeatedly being used and rejected. As a woman I carried this broken little girl who tried everything to be loved and accepted by her village. That little girl developed so much anger and self-hate. I carried hurtful secrets and I was the victim who was often blamed for my own victimization. Toxic villages can create childhood issues that later serve as the foundation for deep-seated adult insecurities.

Being raised in the church as the child of a preacher, I watched my father and my mother work tirelessly. My father with his love for the youth ministry and my mother with her love for the women's ministry gave the church a lot of their time. They were powerful spiritually with the church at heart; ministering and willingly helping those they knew meant them no good. Being a preacher's child was emotionally draining as it exposed me to so much ridicule and judgment. I carried the heavy burdens of other's expectations and opinions. I felt like I lived my life in the spotlight of others' expectations and in the shadows of my parents' ministry; there was no margin of error. I wasn't afforded any mercy living in the shadows of my parents' ministry.

I was told from the time I was a little girl how gifted I was and how God had anointed me for a greater purpose. I grew up at the altar learning to pray and reverence God, but I also learned about the dark underbelly of the church. I learned to both love and despise the church. I fought my calling and the traditions the church stood on. Although at times I rebelled, I must admit, knowing God saved me from situations that would have destroyed me.

As an adult, I carried those childhood traumas, but I learned to mask them. I strived to obtain success to validate my own self-worth. I tried to distance myself from that little girl. But little did I know, those seeds they planted would continue to grow like weeds in a field attempting to suffocate any good vegetation. Those labels followed me, so did the fear of being rejected. I detached emotionally forgetting how to create true emotional attachment. I wore my mask so well no one saw the brokenness, just the anger. I clinched my secrets close to my bosom, never to be spoken.

I carried feelings of rejection, loneliness, abandonment, despair, hopelessness, and worthlessness. I felt like I was losing on every turn. As soon as I thought things were getting better, I would be ambushed. All I wanted was someone to see that goodness within me. It just seemed like I could never stop fighting! My entire life has always been a fight, a struggle.

Finally, I was married, in law school, and had the family I always imagined I would have, but then my health failed me. The doctors had given me up. I was placed on life support and my family was told to say their farewells. As I lay in the hospital after surviving what the doctors thought I would not, I realized the life I once knew was no more. The first man I had completely opened myself to, closed himself to me. My marriage was failing. I felt like he despised the thought of having a sickly wife to care for. I looked in the mirror not knowing who that woman was staring back at me.

My life was not looking anything like God promised me it would. At that point in my life my spirituality became a burden, and a source of pain and confusion. I was praying, and everything was still falling apart. I was at a low point and God obviously wasn't listening to me. I was angry with God and what He allowed. I felt I had angered God and was being punished. I hadn't realized I'd completely lost my identity. I had no identity outside being a mother, sister, daughter, and being a wife. The only other identity I had was being an attorney, but I struggled to pass the bar exam. The emotions I had never allowed myself to feel were boiling over. I was pushed to a point of complete brokenness.

I was in a very dark place void of emotion where I was sure I could not recover from. Amazingly, it was in my brokenness I was able to find wholeness. It was in chaos I finally found the peace I had been seeking for years. I had looked for things in people, expected people to provide things that could only come from within myself. I realized that little girl in me had to be healed and take accountability and that's when the soul searching began.

In my journey to self-discovery and healing, I realized it was inevitable for things to occur in life. It was my response to those things that truly made the difference between building a life of peace and prosperity or leaving it in shambles. I had to learn every failure wasn't life defining. Every mistake wasn't to be carried like a badge of shame, but a learning tool. Moving forward isn't always easy, because it requires taking responsibility for the role you played in your own downfall.

In life I dwelled on the hurts, the mistakes, and the failures. I dwelled in my place of failure not realizing moving forward was essential. It is your process. It is your walk. You must go through it. You must be at peace with the life you have built. Learning those lessons almost destroyed me.

However, God did not allow my destruction. My journey to healing has not been an easy one, but each day I get one step closer to wholeness — mind, body and soul. I spent so much time fighting for acceptance, love, and attention. I found happiness when I learned to fight for myself. I found freedom when I learned to forge my own path.

We spend so much time fighting for everything and everyone else, we neglect to fight for ourselves. We lose ourselves in other's battles creating painful cycles. At some point we must stop, reset, and re-think the course of our lives. Some of us accomplish that on our own and some of us life forces it upon us. I have come through many battles scarred, but victorious. I have come through many battles defeated and deflated, but I continued to fight.

My favorite scripture Jeremiah 29:11 says, "for I know the plans I have for you, declares the Lord, plans to prosper you and not harm you, plans to give you hope and a future." That is the assurance that no matter what I lost, there was a plan that included something greater for me. I just had to trust in the process and FIGHT!

# JOURNEY TO HEALING

Life often forces us to review our lives, our hurts, the people we have hurt, our disappointments, our successes, our failures, and the choices we have made. In the end you are better for it. This exercise is designed to help start the reflection and start the healing.

1. Journaling is a great way to get your thoughts out. But for it to work, one must be honest with themselves.

2. What does the ideal version of yourself look like?

    a. Who are you?

    _____

    _____

    _____

    _____

    b. What are your best attributes?

    _____

    _____

    _____

    _____

c. What are your weaknesses?

_____

_____

_____

_____

d. What are your strengths?

_____

_____

_____

_____

3. What goals did you set for yourself? Why weren't they accomplished?

_____

_____

_____

_____

a. Look at your failures
b. Look at the cause of your failures — even if it was you

  c. Look at your successes and what made them a success

4. This may be one of the hardest, what labels have been placed on you that has made being "you" difficult? What mask have you been wearing? What is that mask covering up?

All my life I have had to deal with people

_____

which has made it difficult to truly be who I am. I have been placed in a box that demanded I _____

_____.

For years I have masked my hurt and my disappointments by _____

_____.

The first step on the journey to healing is to acknowledge you are broken.

I was raised in a small town in South Carolina. I was the fourth child, the only girl, of my parents, however my father had two other children. I was always a dreamer. I felt like I was so much more than a small-town girl. I graduated from USC-Upstate in Spartanburg, South Carolina with a degree in Criminal Justice. I went on to pursue a Master's in Business and Human Resource Development from Webster University in Columbia, South Carolina. While working on my second master's degree, I gave birth to my first child. His birth came at a pivotal moment in my life. He was born two weeks after my mother passed. Shortly after giving birth to him, I was accepted into the Charleston School of Law.

While in law school, I had my second child. That same year I was diagnosed with Lupus Nephritis which almost ended my life. I had to take a year off from school due to being hospitalized. I recovered, returned to school, and graduated with my Juris Doctorate in 2013. In 2020, I founded the nonprofit, See Me the Fighting Butterfly: A Journey to Healing. This organization is to bring awareness of the struggles of those diagnosed with a chronic disease and the effect on the family unit. It was also founded to provide education, support and encouragement to those dealing with the effects of such a diagnosis.

# PAIN POSITIONED ME FOR PURPOSE
## TERE'SA GORHAM

*D*on't let failure talk you out of your future. Have you ever asked yourself why? Why am I going through this and what did I do to deserve this? God is this really the road I have to travel? I'm Teresa Gorham, a 44-year-old single mother of three. I am a Licensed Cosmetologist and Educator who has been in the field for over 26 years. I have been mentored and trained under some amazing, well qualified instructors. Being able to outlive the labels that people have put on you comes with a determination to work on your mindset and a willingness to be free from it. Negative spoken words enter into your ear gate, then your mind for processing, then settles in your heart where it can become locked in. It causes you to be a prisoner of your own mind while causing a war within you. *"God help me! God free me! God Give me the keys and the strategies to break free!"*

For me it wasn't limited to the labels that were put on me but more about the ones that I put on myself. I would say things to myself like: *"Girl, you failed!"* *"What are you gonna do now?" "They're looking at you!" "Maybe they don't need what you have to offer?" "I wonder which story they got about you that isn't true." "Will I ever recover?" "I let my family down!" "Girl, how you gonna bounce back?"*

In 2009, with the help of my dad (God rest his soul) and my mom, I opened my first storefront hair salon business. It was my time and God was blessing. My startup cost was over $30,000 in cash and bartering services. I knew how to grind and hustle with my eyes closed, blocking out all that wasn't contributing to this goal! So excited and eager, my faith was on 100. I only had one month's rent for the building in the bank and I decided that I was going to take a chance. So, with much prayer and desire that's what I did! I opened the salon I always wanted. Even with the pressures of being a single mom it was always my goal to be better for my children. I pushed, and I accomplished. This was the most exciting time in my career!

Being able to operate and have full control over my passion and God-given gift was amazing. That is until what I call "The Interruption" happened. Sometimes interruptions come to distract you from your purpose and the direction in which you should stay! In an effort to assist a "friend", I made an unhealthy business decision to purchase their business, which in turn caused me to uproot my business and move to another part of town. A business deal that was supposed to be good for both parties. This was a heart move and not a prayerful move! From this I learned that every decision that you make has a voice, and it's up to you to listen and hear.

Proverbs 4:6 (TPT) says, "Stick with wisdom and she will stick with you, protecting you throughout your days.

She will rescue all those who passionately listen to her voice." The heart will have you to make an emotional decision that can be hard to recover from. A decision that feels good but may not be good for you! You tend to make moves with good intentions based on the people and surrounding circumstances. This heart move caused me to lose over $15,000 in set up fees and business expenses. By purchasing this business and assisting a "friend" during their business transition to another state, I lost money and someone I called a friend! Psalms 55:20 (TPT) says, "I was betrayed by my friend, though I live in peace with him. While he was stretching out his hand of friendship, he was secretly breaking every promise he had ever made."

Pause — note to self:

- Oil and water don't mix (personal and business) — keep business, business period!
- Slow down and think! Process what's going on.
- Consult accountable people in business before making big moves.
- Learn how to say no! Especially if you are unsure

I'm telling my story, my testimony because God allowed things in my life to crumble and fall apart in plain sight for everyone one to see, but because my DNA make up is to eat the cookie crumbs, it was hard to see the cookies falling apart in my life. I said, *"God Why Me?"*

I had to close my business. That day was a numbing feeling and I chose not to feel that day! I never even expressed outwardly my emotions at that point. That day I was not going to deal with the matters of the heart, so I asked myself, *"Girl what is your next move?"* My clients were important to me, so I had to think fast!

I wasn't behind in rent at my second location. I made sure the rent at the salon was paid but couldn't pay my rent at home. My business was being sabotaged and was under attack and I didn't even know it. There was so much talk in the street unbeknownst to me. My "friend" that sold me her business and moved out of state, was now flying in town every month just 5 months after selling me the business, and she decided to rent a salon chair on the same block as me. She didn't even tell me or call but I heard it from a few honest customers that received a call to come back to her for services. I was crushed! I was hurt because she was my friend, but this was business as some would say. Imagine! No one knew the domino effect that was happening. It put me in a compromising position. Lord knows I only want the best for people so how could this happen?

Labels rang in my ear: *"Girl you're a failure!" "How did you let your dream fail?" "Why did you move your salon?" "You should've said no."* Meanwhile, the lights were getting cut off at home and my gas was on a payment plan about to be cut off. But I couldn't break! I couldn't. I had babies that had to eat! I lost my apartment, not once but twice all while owning my business and going to work every day. Only close family and friends knew. It all happened so fast! I still kept my head up believing in God, and always got dressed and put my face on. I was about to just give up and move to North Carolina with my parents and just start all over. In my mind I said, *"It ain't worth it. Just take your babies and leave."* My worth seemed unredeemable in that moment. I told myself, *"They don't show you no love anyway!"* No honor in your own dwelling place! Labels. Labels I put on myself and voices of failure flooded my mind, but God had me covered.

I opened a salon suite which I also had to close, but I was pushing! I pushed so hard even when I closed my salons, but I never missed a beat doing hair. I cried, "God! God! Say this ain't so..." I decided to stay with a great friend for three months and finally regained my fight. When I moved out I was ready, and I've been fighting ever since! Somethings happen in your life not only to make you aware but to also prepare you to help others. The love of God has covered me, and forgiveness has been key in my healing process. Psalm 32:10 (TPT) says, "So my conclusion is this: Many are the sorrows and frustrations of those who don't come clean with God. But when you trust in the Lord for forgiveness his wrap-around love will surround you."

God is still writing my story, I continue to operate as a Licensed Cosmetologist and CEO of DimensionsBy TeresaG.Com, an online Hair Extensions Company. I am currently one of the Lead Cosmetology Instructors for an Inner-City Non-Profit Program in Connecticut, and currently enrolled in an online certification program at Harvard for Business in Emerging Economies. Forgiveness is key to a journey of healing. You, too, can overcome and win! Say to yourself "I WILL WIN!"

1. Make a list of labels that people have put on you.

_____

_____

_____

_____

_____

2. Make a list of labels that you have put on yourself.

_____

_____

_____

_____

_____

3. Read these labels out loud and denounce them. Taking their power away and **X** them out as you go along. Then ask God for forgiveness and healing if you have ever operated within any of these labels.

_____

_____

_____

_____

_____


4. Now make a list of positive labels that describe you and/or list labels that describe the person you are becoming.

_____

_____

_____

_____

_____


5. Read them to yourself day, make copies or post it as a reminder of reasons you desire to win.

_____

_____

_____

_____

_____

Tere'sa S. Gorham is a native of Norwalk, CT and CEO of Dimensionsbyteresag.com. With over 25 years of experience in the hair industry and over 6 years as a salon owner, Tere'sa has built a strong reputation in hair weaving and non-medical hair replacement. Her innovative hair styles have been displayed in various events across the Tri-State area.

In 2014, Tere'sa's strong desire to educate and mentor new stylist and salon owners, led her to develop a hairweaving workshop called "Back to the Basic". In 2017, she continued to push boundaries by launching Dimensionsbyteresag.com, a top selling hair extension and hair care company. Tere'sa continues to break barriers by growing her online hair business and devoting her time to educating inner city youth at a nonprofit agency in Bridgeport, CT.

Not a stranger to education herself, Tere'sa sharpened her skills by becoming a Certified Cranial Prosthetic Specialist. She is currently enrolled in Harvardx's certification course, "Entrepreneurship in Emerging Economies."

https://www.dimensionsbyteresag.com/
Dimensions by Ter'esa G - Home (facebook.com)
Dimensions by Teresa G (@dimensionsbyteresag)

# EMOTIONAL TRAUMA
## A GOLIATH IN THE MIND
### KEISHA EDWARDS

*D*o you ever wonder why head wounds bleed the most? The brain requires a tremendous amount of blood-flow to maintain the work of driving the vehicle of your body. I pray the blood of Jesus will flow through your mind, renew every pathway of your mind that has been affected by trauma, and transform you into a new creature by the words of my testimony. One of my childhood memories was seeing my dad physically abuse my mother in the bathroom of our home in Jamaica. I remember the bathroom being a neon green with a craw-foot white tub. The bathroom wasn't complete because as a child we lived in a house that wasn't finished because my dad was still fixing it up while we lived in the two front rooms. It's funny how as a child your spiritual senses are so in tune. I don't remember my dad at that moment; all I saw was a monster. I had to be pretty small, because I remember he was huge in my little eyes. In that moment I truly knew what FEAR was. The fear was a crippling monster and it was in my daddy. The emotional trauma began for me that very moment. Fear entered my heart like a serpent. Although it meant to cut off the very air I breathe, God had another plan.

I was always a very smart child and book smarts came very easily to me. I went almost a whole year of skipping days of school and brought home on my report card close to straight A's. My father wasn't aware, because I would come home and steal the mail out of the mailbox. When my father did find out it was about a year later and he got so mad that he sent me to Jamaica. I wasn't able to return to America unless I wrote him a letter of apology. At that time, I was a very stubborn teenager, so it took about a year for me to write the apology. Meanwhile, I got pregnant with my daughter at the age of 16. After writing the apology he allowed me to come back to America and when I returned I found out I was pregnant. My heavenly father knew that I needed something in my life to steer me off the road that I was leading on, and that was my child. On the other hand, my earthly father was livid with me and sent me to England to live with my mom. I had to return to the U.S. every six months because I was a U.S. resident. I would travel to America and stay for a short time and then return to England with my mom.

I remember traveling back to England and a strong sensation from the pit of my soul took over me. I had a feeling that something was going to happen to my dad and I was going to be too far away. That sensation never left, and it was overwhelming as a teenager. I didn't know how to deal with it, so I just suppressed it and disconnected from it. Months later my family called and told us that my dad had died. That sensation that I couldn't shake for months was like a plug hitting a socket! It overwhelmed me, and I cried for days. I felt like I was having an out-of-body experience looking at myself crying. My mom tried to console me, but her voice just got further and further away. I believe that was my first experience with the power of God. I believe God was showing me that there was something out there that was bigger than me.

Fear overtook me! I was unaware of the possession that fear had in my life. I lived in survival mode for many years. In survival mode you're not worried about sowing the right seeds, you're just surviving to remain alive and existing with no purpose. I would often say that I had to survive and couldn't dwell on the things that happened to me. I didn't want those things to dictate my life! In reality fear was dictating everything. Everything I would try to do I would be crippled. As soon as trials came my way I would stop my education, my goals, and my dreams. I would find a reason why I couldn't finish or accomplish them. Thoughts of fear would bombard my mind and I was unable to complete my divine purpose. In survival mode I could only maintain being a mom and holding a job. I gave all of myself to my child and put my desires on the back burner. Although I didn't know who I was or whose I was my destiny was still written. It will come to fruition because God will complete what He starts.

I was 17 years old when my dad died. My daughter had just turned one and we were on the plane to Jamaica to bury my dad. A few years later my youngest brother was brutally murdered at the age of 18. I remember the day that I was told that he died. I worked at UPS and it was one of those weeks that you couldn't wait to end. I remember saying, "I just can't wait until Friday gets here." The power of your words! It's amazing that we don't live in the present; always wanting to move to the next moment not knowing what it brings. On Friday my whole world turned upside down. I heard the news while coming out of work; they thought my brother was dead in a shooting. I couldn't imagine him being in a shooting because he wasn't that kind of kid. He was still a little nerdy kid that grew up during the summer. I remember going to the site where the incident took place.

While waiting for hours for someone to tell us if my brother was alive or dead I remember how I knew he was gone. I saw the shirt that he wore the night before in the police officer's hand and I knew. My heart was just so broken! I didn't know how to process what I was seeing and hearing. My baby brother was gone, and it wasn't just one murder it was two. I also lost my cousin on that day. I felt like life was slipping through my fingers and I didn't know how to move from that moment. How much can one person bear? I was his big sis and I didn't protect him. I couldn't breathe. All I felt was death and my very existence was death. I was lost in a mass of unsolved emotions. Someone unlocked the flood gates and there was a mess at my feet. I needed help!

Fear had overtaken me again. The awareness of fear and its possession in my life was evident. Survival is the state or the fact of continuing to exist. I was just existing! I would wake up, go to work, and repeat. The devil had me on an orbiting cycle that turned on its own axis. My life was in a cycle of just existing and never truly walking in purpose. My heart was broken. The traumas I experienced in my life dictated my every decision. Fear consumed my choices, but God was working out all my trials and my tribulations for my good.

Years later I met a woman on my job who invited me to church. From that moment God took me on a journey of renewing my mind. He uprooted the seeds of the enemy and planted the seeds of His living word. He continues to show me that through every trial, every tribulation, and every trauma He was always with me. He has molded and shaped me for His purpose to tell my testimony and reach every broken-hearted, every emotionally traumatized, and every rejected soul that crosses my path and tell them about a man named Jesus. He can deliver you out of dark places, renew your mind, and set you free to take back His kingdom.

Keisha Edwards is a native of Kingston, Jamaica and was raised in Silver Springs, Maryland. She is a loving mother who works in dialysis in the healthcare field. She is a powerful woman of God that loves the Lord. Her godly purpose is to rid His people of the toxins of the devil through the power of the Holy Spirit and bring his people back in right standing with Him and not just experience His Power, but dwell in the reservoir of His very existence. Keisha is a published author and resides in East Hartford, Connecticut.

# POETICALLY AND UNAPOLOGETICALLY ME

## NATASHA GORHAM

*So, you want to call me black, tar-baby, and ugly?*
*Don't laugh, I don't think any of that was funny.*
*Didn't you know that I was a shade of you?*
*When God created man,*
*His image was of me and of you?*
*Don't be upset because you seem to be confused.*
*Didn't you know that I was a shade of you?*
*NSG – Shades of You c.1999*

For as long as I can remember, there has been a label, from one facet to another. If it wasn't about my looks, then it was about my size. If it wasn't about my size, then it was about my color. If it wasn't about my color, then it was about something else like common sense, or even plain ignorance. As much as I say it, I truly do care, and words hurt — they can get you even when you think they are not there. Creeping up on you in moments of despair, reminding you, *"Hey girl, hey boy – look I'm right here."* And what do hurt people do? They go on a mission to make others feel what they are hiding inside, all the while destroying who they can with their mean and nasty oral vibes, and that is just how it can be.

Labels don't define me. I am who I am, unapologetically. I can't place my story from a single situation (you'll have to grab one of my books and a nice cup of tea to understand what made me, simply me). But to be frank, there is a story of where all of this began. I am a petite, seasoned lady with a large family. Many times, I have hidden in shame, holding onto my secrets and inner pain. But to others they see my strength, but out of routine I survived the struggles because I gave everything my best. That was my habit.

One of my temple rubs would be the phrase, *"There she goes... the one with all of those kids!"* I truly dislike being spoken about in that manner, because there is so much more to me than, "just having a bunch of kids." Honestly having babies was the furthest thing from my mind, but they are here and by golly, they are mine and I love them and anyone else's if you really need to know. There was a time when the doctors told me that I'll never have any more kids. It saddened me to the core and made me feel less than a woman. See, I struggled too. I cried so much, I was so sad and blue. But in that sadness, God allowed them to come through. So, they are my miracle kids, and it can happen for you too! I have not one regret behind it. And ladies guess what, with half of my girly parts – that's how God did it! So again, I chose to keep every one of my blessings. And if that is your struggle, keep trusting! I'm so glad I had all of my babies young, because one day I went to the doctor and was diagnosed with an illness that will now prevent me from having more children. So, you see, don't judge anyone's walk because you don't have all the information behind the scenes. My babies are all amazing, they are so important to me, and we are doing just fine. My little legacies remind me each day to simply just smile. Not every day is easy, but we seem to be doing alright. And yes, I do have help.

To the single mother, yes you can do it on your own. There will be struggles and hardships, but if that is your choice, there are things you should know. A father's touch means so much, so no matter how you feel about that man, at the end of the day, that is still his kid. It took two to create the miracle you chose to push through, so get over yourself and your feelings and stop holding kids as hostages or using them as leverage. Ask me how I know? Life taught me a lesson and now I know what I know. Would I do things differently? Not really – I'm still healing and dealing. But if your situation allows, find a place in your heart to understand and accept the fact that baby boys and baby girls need that loving touch from a man. Allow each other to help raise your child. Do it amicably and please be loving and kind. There are too many damaged individuals running around with Mommy and Daddy issues. Make the change and mature gracefully.

To that person who's insecure, what is all of that self-hate for? No one can define beauty. Beauty can be anything and no baby, you are not ugly. Put your shoulders back, stand tall, walk that walk, and break that wall. Remember nobody can do it better than you, wear your confidence and come through. So what if your parents didn't instill confidence in you, did you know that you've *still* got this? Find some confidence and do it quickly. Never let others make you feel less than yourself, if they got something to say, politely say next, willfully!

To that person struggling with an illness, I feel your pain, but you must find the strength and will to conquer this hardship each day. There is sunshine after all that rain. Push to find the will to prosper, the will to survive. Your illness does not make you, you can and will be alright and guess what, if you're reading this — newsflash, you're still alive. Your illness can, and never will define the amazing person that you are. People may not understand your situation, and that is ok. There is absolutely, positively, no reason to explain. Finally, to the person who is dealing with grief and/or hurt. You've got this and trust me, faith really works. God can soothe your troubling pain, just take things day by day. You are not the first and not the last. Better days are coming, just keep looking ahead. Time makes things alright but go ahead and cry if that is what you need to do to get through those dark nights.

I could go on and on but just know my faith has kept me strong. It is that mustard seed, the speckle of something that cannot be seen. I challenge God where He is, and remind Him, "Hey, Daddy, I'm still your kid!" There is no secret and really no road map, everyone's walk is different but there are similarities to all of that. Trust the process and be strong each day, but amidst all of this don't forget to pray. I'm no one famous, just some regular old girl, trying to make her mark in this here world. I have nothing flashy, just a whole lot of love and encouragement to give. Be blessed, as I am still a whole piece of work in progress.

## Activity

### Understanding Your Trauma

Look, I've been through a lot, but my hurts and pains are NOT your invitation to abuse me, add stress or drama, or hurt to what I've already been through. We have all been through things, but it is my duty to not allow the very things that I have been through to affect you or anyone else for that matter. I must deal with my things and my baggage, so I am accountable of being a kind and good human being to others. But we all have "OUR DAYS." So how do I get to that place? I OWN IT! So, let's trigger this trauma and force these feelings to go.

Quickly, grab a pen and paper. (I'll wait, because I am grabbing mine as I am writing this to you). Great, now think of one thing that triggers you and upsets you to the core. It could be something that you have carried and has weighed you down. Do you have it? Ok, good. Now on that piece of paper – write to that thing. Let it all out. Give that paper your all – put it all on there. Tell that thing how you really feel. Go on, don't be shy. This is your chance and opportunity to give it all you've got.

Now that you have poured it all out, let's pray: "*God we come to you as humbly as we know how thanking you and praising you for another day. Lord if anything in my heart is not like you, please take it out as I need you this very hour. Today I ask that you give me the strength and courage to release this very thing that has bothered me and heal my troubled heart. Help me to find peace and replace that emptiness and sadness with love, happiness and your amazing joy. Mend my broken heart and allow me to continue to be free. Give me the strength and courage to release this thing so it no longer bothers me. God, I give this pain to you and I am excited for the strength to help me to get over this mountain in my life. As of today, this trauma will not trigger me. I thank you and praise you for my road to being complete. In Jesus Name I pray, Amen."*

Now listen, you can pray how you pray, that was just an example of what I would say in my personal prayer. You can decide to destroy the paper or hold onto it, but now that it's out – let that thing GO!

Unpacking these things can be hard because it causes you to relive some things that you wanted to keep buried deep. Teach your kids not to bury things, release and break those cycles to become free. Don't harbor ill feelings but season your tongue and express yourself in a calm manner respectfully and peacefully. Life is way too short to hold grudges, so if you've offended anyone be the bigger person and apologize. If they offended you forgive and be free. Find your peace and reclaim it back. I wish you all amazing success and bountiful blessings. Be bold, be beautiful. But most importantly: Be You – Undefined.

Thank you for sharing this time.

❦

Natasha S. Gorham is a graduate of the University of Bridgeport where she was featured on the Dean's List, numerous Honor Societies, as well as Student of the Year. With a heart of helping as many people as she can, she finds time to be a mother to her children as well as helping to assist and guide others. Currently she spends her time reading and writing as well as being a Lupus Advocate for which she enjoys bringing awareness to the disease. Loved by many, she is a joy to have as a sister and friend in multiple people's lives. Currently she is working on a solo project that is coming soon. You can find her on Instagram at beyoutifully_undefined or visit her webpage at www.beyoutifullyundefined.com where she is inspiring individuals to just simply Be U!

Thank you for supporting *Outlive the Labels Volume II*!

If you learned anything from this book or found it helpful, we'd be very grateful if you would post a short review on Amazon. Your support does make a difference!

To leave a review, simply type in "Outlive the Labels Volume II: From Trauma to Triumph on Amazon" in the search bar of your internet browser, and the link to Amazon will show up.

If you would like to be a future co-author of an Outlive the Labels book project, please email info@marykayeholmes.com

Thank you again for your support.